THE
TEEN FACE
BOOK

A Question and Answer Guide to Skin Care, Cosmetics, and Facial Plastic Surgery

Prepared by the
American Academy of
Facial Plastic and
Reconstructive Surgery

ACROPOLIS BOOKS LTD.
WASHINGTON, D.C.

ACROPOLIS BOOKS LTD.

Alphons J. Hackl, Founder
Colortone Building
2400 17th St. NW
Washington, DC 20009

Attention: Schools and Corporations
ACROPOLIS books are available at quantity discounts with bulk purchase for educational, business, or sales promotional use. For information, please write to: SPECIAL SALES DEPARTMENT, ACROPOLIS BOOKS LTD., 2400 17th St. NW, Washington, DC 20009.

Are there Acropolis books you want but cannot find in your local stores?
You can get any Acropolis book title in print. Simply send title and retail price. Be sure to add postage and handling: $2.25 for orders up to $15.00; $3.00 for orders from $15.01 to $30.00; $3.75 for orders over $100.00. District of Columbia residents add applicable sales tax. Enclose check or money order only, no cash please, to:

ACROPOLIS BOOKS LTD.
2400 17th St. NW
WASHINGTON, DC 20009

Library of Congress Cataloging-in-Publication Data

```
The Teen face book : a Q&A guide to looking your best
  /prepared by the American Academy of Facial Plastic and
  Reconstructive Surgery.  p. cm.
  Summary:  Discusses various types of facial plastic
surgery such as removal of birthmarks, reconstruction after
injuries, and jaw realignment.
  ISBN 0-87491-957-6  :  $12.95
  1.  Face--Surgery--Miscellanea.  2.  Teenagers--Surgery--
Miscellanea.  3.  Surgery, Plastic--Miscellanea.  [1.  Face-
Surgery.  2.  Surgery.  Plastic--Miscellanea.]  I.  American
Academy of Facial  RD119.5.F33&68 1989
617.5'20592--dc20                                89-17908
                                                    CIP
                                                    AC
```

Cover Photo: By Rhoda Baer. Front row from left: John Anthony Cangemi, Aveek Nath, Melanie Jones, and Christina Roe. Back row, from left: Carrie Autumn Worsley, Jennifer Lloyd, and Jamie Lee Cool. These teen models were selected for their individual style and have not necessarily had facial plastic surgery.

Contents

Preface:
'I Like the Way I Look'

Tracey had always hated her nose. "I would never consider going out without makeup on," she recalls. "I did everything to try and cover it up, and I never let people see my profile. But the nose really defines the face, and when you have a nose like mine was, there is really no way to hide it."

No matter how she tried to disguise her nose, Tracey remained extremely self-conscious. "I was upset every time I looked in the mirror," she says. "My nose wasn't a deformity, exactly, but in my eyes it was very unattractive."

From the time she was 14, Tracey knew she would seek a permanent solution to her problem—facial plastic surgery. Although some teens may consider facial plastic surgery a rather drastic solution, for Tracey, who lives in suburban New York City, it was not unusual. "You have to understand that cosmetic surgery is very popular here. For girls between the ages of 14 and 20, having a rhinoplasty [nasal surgery] is not a rare thing." At first Tracey's parents didn't agree. They felt she looked just fine. "But they knew how I felt about my nose, and once they understood I was determined to have the surgery, they supported me 100 percent." They all agreed she would wait until she was 17 to have the surgery.

Two years after her surgery, Tracey remains enthusiastic. "The biggest change has been in my personality. Before the surgery I was inhibited and shy because I always thought people were looking at my nose. Today I like the way I look, so I'm more outgoing." Tracey notes that she read a great deal about how to improve her appearance before deciding to have surgery. That is essential, she and other patients feel, to understanding exactly what can be accomplished with a cosmetic makeover or a new hairstyle—and what may be correctable only through facial plastic surgery.

Tracey says she wishes she had had a book that explained all the options, and it is that same wish, multiplied many times by young people and parents across the country, that led to the writing of *The Teen Face Book: A Question and Answer Guide to Skin Care, Cosmetics, and Facial Plastic Surgery.*

The authors are members of the world's largest association of facial plastic surgeons, the American Academy of Facial Plastic and Reconstructive Surgery. A major focus of our work is to help young people make educated choices about ways they can improve their appearance and thereby increase their self-confidence. We hope this book will help you sort out your feelings about your appearance, find ways to enhance your natural look, and, if facial plastic surgery is your ultimate choice, understand what you realistically might expect from each surgical procedure available to teens today.

Introduction:

Looking Good Is Feeling Great

When Kathleen, 15, cut short a vacation in California to return to her hometown in Kansas for a chance to model in a hair salon video, she found herself left standing on the sidelines. "We're sorry," she was told, "but we already have a blonde with your 'look.'"

Penny, 16, found the courage to audition for a slot on the cheerleading squad even though she was overweight and considered unattractive by her peers. She wasn't booed, exactly, but when the student body voted, Penny was at the bottom of the list.

John, 17, another Midwesterner, tried to get a job to save money for college by applying to several fast food operations. He's convinced he was turned down each time because of the length of his hair. A friend who works at a fast food restaurant on the East Coast points out that it's the good-looking kids who are put on the front line, manning the cash registers and taking orders. Employees who aren't so attractive are stationed back at the grill.

"At our school, parking lot assignments were decided by the student body president, who was a guy," confides Terry, 16. "All the paved parking spaces went to the pretty girls and to his buddies."

Face it. In today's culture, looks *do* count, especially for teens. Whether it's a modeling job or just a date for the senior prom, your appearance is on the line. You may wish that society was less judgmental, but you have to accept that how you look affects how people relate to you—and often how you relate to them.

"Everyone knows that the good-looking guys don't date ugly girls or girls who are fat," points out Susan, age 15.

"Student Council and especially Homecoming Court—these people are always chosen for their looks, not their personality," comments Jennifer, 17.

"Often the teacher will walk into a class on the first day and decide by your looks how he will treat you for the entire year," maintains Sean, 16.

Many teens understandably are dismayed with this focus on looks, even as they acknowledge it exists. "What in history has caused mankind to put so much emphasis on looks?" laments Joel, 17. "Whatever happened to inner beauty?" Another young man, age 16, comments, "People shouldn't be that concerned with their facial features. We shouldn't allow people to make us feel inferior because of them." "I always try my best to look good," says Sara, 14, "but I sure wish looks weren't that important."

Of the more than two hundred teens interviewed for this book, nearly all know at least one friend or classmate who is not particularly attractive but, because he or she has a classy personality or witty sense of humor, is a lot of fun to be with. These individuals have gone beyond their looks and have, as one teen bluntly remarked, "broken the ugly barrier."

"There are many unattractive people I like for their personality," acknowledges Dianna, 14. *"A smile and a sense of humor go a long way in making friends."*

Carey, 17, notes, "I know a girl who isn't pretty at all. She has a very crooked nose. People call her names and laugh, but she laughs right along with them. She has a great attitude toward life."

"The wittiest boy in our class is also the ugliest," notes David, 14. "I think he is very bold and courageous."

It also is true that "beauty is in the eye of the beholder." Often a person will worry about some detail of his or her appearance that others don't even notice. It's easy for a young person to begin worrying more and more about a facial "blemish" that actually is perfectly normal. Before you start worrying about your facial features, take a minute to look at others your age who are popular. Chances are, most of them don't have "perfect" features.

Further inspiration are the young people who have become quite successful in the entertainment world despite obvious appearance liabilities. Some of the most popular stars are what might be considered too short or too plain for stardom. Many rock stars have become quite successful despite their less-than-classic looks.

Looks that are too perfect can be a liability, too. Both guys and girls feel that the best looking of their classmates often let it go to their head. Such individuals frequently are accused of acting stuck-up or snobbish.

"I'm really suspicious if a guy who is too good-looking asks me out," comments Karen, 19. *"That intimidates me. I wonder why he's doing it."*

"A friend of mine actually lost a job because she was too pretty," relates Susan, 15. *"The boss didn't want a lot of guys hanging around."*

Focus on Looks Not All Bad

At first glance, this emphasis on appearance seems superficial and vain, but on second analysis it may not be all bad.

The point to looking your best, says psychologist Dr. Joyce Brothers, is to be able to forget about yourself and be self-confident. "When you look good and feel great, people treat you as if you're special," she says. "Your appearance sends signals to others about who you are, how you feel, even about your values and aspirations. When people treat you as if you are intelligent and friendly, you behave that way, and that starts an upward spiral of success."

FOR BETTER OR FOR WORSE LYNN JOHNSTON

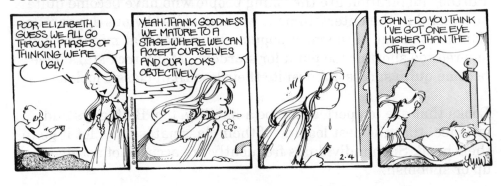

Other psychologists, too, regard a little vanity as a good thing. Attention to one's looks is a sign of self-esteem, just as lack of interest in grooming and appearance is an early sign of depression. Thus, appearance has a lot to do with how you feel about yourself, both inside and outside. It helps to shape your self-image.

"If I feel I look good in the morning, then I feel good all day long," points out Amy, 19, speaking for a lot of her peers.

"When I look at myself in the mirror, I see an average-looking person," says Marcy, 16. "If my acne is bad at the time or I just don't look my best, I tend to be in a bad mood or depressed about my looks. If I look good, I'm in a better mood and I feel good and confident about myself."

"I have a friend whose mood and self-confidence depend entirely on how his hair looks. If his hair was cut to the middle of his neck without his knowledge, it is safe to say his self-confidence would all but disappear and his mood would shift from arrogant to withdrawn and extremely shy," notes Marc, 19.

Looking Good Takes Time

It is no secret that young people spend a great deal of time working at looking good. And it's perfectly healthy and normal to try to make the best of your appearance.

As Lisa Sliwa, national director of the Guardian Angels, noted in an interview in *Vogue* magazine, it's balance that counts. "To be obsessed with your appearance is unhealthy. But if you look at improving your physical appearance as part of your overall life strategy, it's empowering."

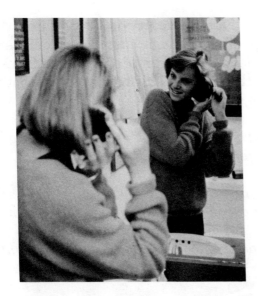

Young people spend a great deal of time on their looks, but experts say that's normal and healthy.

Complexion, hair, and eyes top the list of facial features that most concern guys and girls of all ages. But they have other concerns. Teens want to know how to make their lips look larger — and their noses smaller. They are worried about oily skin, ears that protrude, and the dangers of too much sun. Moles and birthmarks, plump cheeks, and weak chins also cause frustration.

Moreover, despite all of the literature on the subject, teens still aren't sure exactly how drugs, smoking, alcohol, diet, and exercise affect their appearance.

Finding your best look is the subject of the first half of this book. Prompted by questions on health and appearance by hundreds of teens, experts in the fields of beauty, fitness, and medicine share their solutions to everything from acne to hairstyling woes. You'll learn what look is in, and how to achieve the look you want. The trick is to learn how to play up your best features and minimize those that aren't so perfect.

When the Best Cosmetic Tips Are Not Enough

Cosmetics and skincare products expertly used can cover a multitude of facial imperfections. Healthful living, personality, and an inner glow count, too. But there is another option, especially for problems of a more structural nature, and that is facial plastic surgery. For teens in many parts of the country, facial plastic surgery as a cosmetic option is a very new idea.

Rachel, of suburban New York, has several friends who would never think of having cosmetic surgery, and she feels that's great, for them. "But it was the best thing I ever did in my life," she says of her nasal surgery five years ago when she was 13. "It saved me from a future of insecurities."

Toni, 16, who also had facial plastic surgery, acknowledges that focusing on appearance should not be that important. "But I had to be pretty before I could say that."

On the other hand, Jon, 15, says he would never consider surgery unless he was in a disfiguring accident. "We should accept the face we were born with," he maintains.

The point is that facial plastic surgery is a very personal decision. The degree of your facial problem isn't what's important, but how you feel about it is. If your looks bother you on a regular basis, if they are a source of embarrassment or present problems that you cannot address with cosmetics, hairstyle, or other more conventional measures, then facial plastic surgery may be right for you. For a teen whose face has a functional or cosmetic defect from birth, disease, or an accident, facial plastic surgery may be the only answer.

The danger is in believing that facial plastic surgery can change your life. It can't. In fact, the very best facial plastic surgery won't drastically change your looks unless your appearance is quite misshapen to begin with. "When I went to school people knew I looked better, but they didn't exactly know why" is the comment that young facial plastic surgery patients make over and over.

Facial plastic surgery is not for everyone. It won't help you do better in school, and it won't win you friends. In and of itself, it can't get you a boyfriend or girlfriend. But, in some cases, it can help you feel better about yourself, and it can bring out the beauty you feel is hidden inside. For some people, facial plastic surgery relieves worry about appearance so that they can get on with life without focusing obsessively on looks.

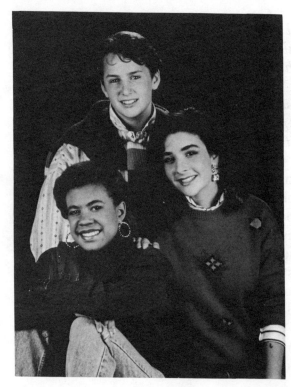

"People who look good usually feel good, thus their outlook on life is more cheerful," says Don, 18. These teens certainly seem proof of that.

I

Looking Different's Not All That Bad

1

Classic Beauty Standards Shape Our Self-image

"There is a girl in my school who is the prettiest of all girls," declares Patti, 17. "She has a perfect classical nose with high cheekbones that accent the oval shape of her face. She has cat-shaped eyes with long curly black eyelashes. Her eyes are deep brown with perfect matching arching eyebrows."

Aspiring teen model Suzanne, 14, admires a more public figure. "Paulina Porizkova [model / Estee Lauder girl] is my ideal," Suzanne enthuses. "She has beautiful skin, expressive eyes, the perfect face—it just seems flawless."

"What can you say about Johnny Depp [actor on '21 Jump Street']?" asks Renee, 16, with a note of awe in her voice. "He is beautiful! He is boyish yet has a maturity about his face."

Classic beauty. Johnny Depp. Paulina Porizkova. Brooke Shields. Tom Cruise. Christie Brinkley.

17

These are the faces we all wish we had been born with, faces that undeniably earn a rating of "10." But what is it about these faces that inspires our admiration and our envy? Why are they "10s"?

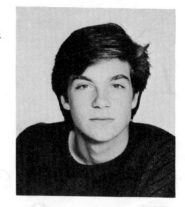

Beauty is often said to be only skin deep. But experts will tell you that true beauty goes clear to the bone. That is because when talking about appearance—either feminine beauty or masculine handsomeness—what really is being discussed is the underlying bone structure. It is the skeleton's proportions, and its angles and contours and curves, that work in harmony to create the concept of beauty.

Jason Bateman's face is cited by many teens as being classically good looking.

The classic beauties have facial structures that follow certain precise mathematical principles. One such principle is that the perfect face can be divided horizontally into equal thirds. To determine your "thirds," use a photograph and divide your face into three sections by drawing horizontal lines through your forehead hairline, your eyebrows, the base of your nose, and the lower edge of your chin. In the ideal face, the three sections are equal (see figure 1).

You also can determine how symmetrical your facial features are by drawing a line from top to bottom through the center of the photograph (see figure 2). Interestingly, human faces are never completely symmetrical. Yet another test of facial balance is to divide your face vertically into equal fifths. The ideal face should be "five eyes wide," that is, five times the width of one eye. The space between your eyes should be the width of one eye. In addition, the width of your nose should not extend beyond the lines drawn down from the inner corners of your eyes (see figure 3).

I've Measured My Face, Now What?

Although you may not have read about the principles of classic beauty, they have shaped western civilization's perception of beauty for more than 2,500 years. They were deduced by the same ancient Greek mathematician, Pythagoras, who devised geometry (and your textbooks) based on his study of the relationships of points, angles, and lines. Today, these principles implicitly guide how we perceive our looks. They subtly influence our selection of cosmetics and hairstyles that emphasize certain features and play down others—a process called *facial sculpting* by cosmeticians. (See chapter 5 for more on cosmetic facial sculpting.)

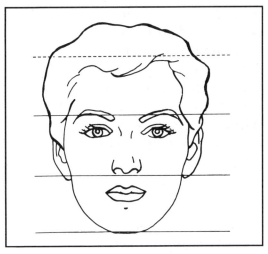

Figure 1: To divide your face into "thirds," draw horizontal lines across your forehead hairline, your brow, the base of your nose, and the lower edge of your chin. In the ideal face, all three sections are equally spaced.

Still, it is well to remember that beauty is in the eye of the beholder. This is fortunate, for it means that not everyone appreciates the same look. "My boyfriend is the best-looking guy I know," says Marlena, 16, who nonetheless is happy that not every girl in her school agrees with her. As the next chapter will reveal, an individual look can be just as sought after as classic beauty.

In deciding the best look for your particular face, you also must take into consideration racial and ethnic differences. Although some beauty consultants advise that the principles of classic proportion hold true regardless of ethnic differences, others believe they pertain primarily to the Caucasian face. Bone structure is different for all races, they note. Skin texture, color, and elasticity vary as well. Whatever the case may be, the point is to find your own look and enjoy it.

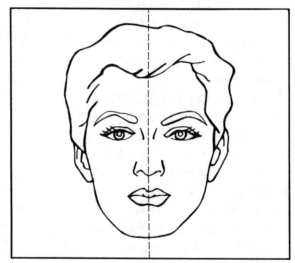

Figure 2: A straight line drawn through the center of your face will show you how symmetrical your features are.

Figure 3: If you divide your face into equal fifths, you can compare it to the classic ideal in which the face is five times the width of one eye. Additionally, the width of your nose should not extend past the inner corners of your eyes.

These figures show one idealized view of "beauty." Although everyone's idea is different, you may find it fun to measure your face using these concepts. But don't worry if your face is not "perfect" —few are.

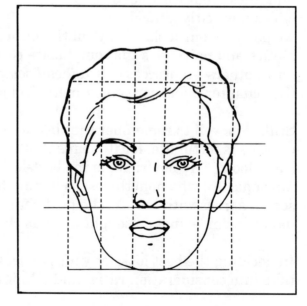

2

The Individual Look Is Predicted for the 1990s

"The best looking girls," declares Tim, 18, "always have a great expression on their face, no matter what."

"High cheekbones, clear tanned skin, long wavy hair, and a full mouth — that's what I think of when I hear 'good-looking,' " reveals Doug, 19.

Joel, 17, focuses on eyes: "The eyes are the most romantic part of the body, truly the windows to the soul. They tell what the person is all about."

Defining good looks is not an easy assignment. Classic bone structure notwithstanding, the concept of beauty changes constantly.

For example, modeling agencies used to insist on the absolutely perfect, classic face. Today, they accept the occasional blemish or imperfection that lends character to a face. *Individuality* is the key word for today's face. A natural look that maintains ethnic characteristics is preferred. In fact, the Click modeling agency in New York City has made its reputation with its unusual and individual looking women. "I'm interested in faces that conjure up thought, humor, integrity," Click's founder, Frances Grill, states.

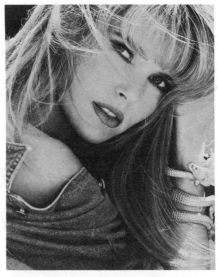

The look that prevailed in fashion modeling for many years — high cheekbones, a thin, almost gaunt appearance — is no longer so popular, points out Mary Ann Van Sickle, a former model and owner of the Models and Images agency in Wichita, Kansas. "High cheekbones do still photograph very well, but everyone doesn't have to have them. When Christie Brinkley came on the scene,

The looks popular in fashion modeling affect current perceptions of beauty. Christie Brinkley's healthy look is the one popular today.

she brought a rounded, healthy look that is more popular today."

The look of the nineties resonates with health and fitness, fashion experts tell us. It's an individual look that doesn't necessarily follow the dictates of the crowd but is a melting pot of styles. For example, New York photographer Steven Meisel says the trend in modeling is a smaller nose, almond-shaped eyes, and full lips. He believes a mix of ethnic and racial characteristics will guide fashion well into the next decade. Katie Ford, creative director of Ford Models in New York, predicts there will be more diversity with no single look declared the ideal.

Such diversity is evident even today. As pressures to conform to the current "in" look have diminished, both sexes have found new freedom to express their inner selves. Model Brooke Shields champions an individual style. "Without a real connection to one's thinking and one's values, one's 'beauty' won't last," commented Shields in a *Vogue* magazine interview. "A positive aspect of feeling good is a more individual approach to one's looks."

"Everyone wants to look different," maintains Carey, 16. "But you have to look really great, too. Your look has to be a positive one."

Brad, 15, agrees. "Nobody really wants to look like everyone else. You don't want to copy someone, but you can pick different looks in people you admire and incorporate them into your own style."

Teens protest that they don't want to look like carbon copy cutouts of everyone else, but they often fail to follow through on their convictions, according to Van Sickle. "They feel a certain identification with a look," Van Sickle says. "It's their security blanket. If the frizzy hair look is in, they all want it. If they see a magazine cover they like, they all want to copy it. It's hard to convince them to accentuate their strong points and develop their own individual look." Girls, it seems, prefer a specific model to emulate while guys prefer a group image. As Jason, 17, puts it, "Guys don't want to

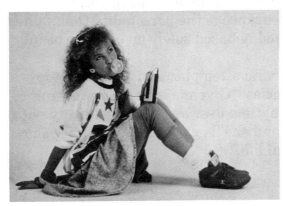

A very individual appearance, as demonstrated by this young woman, is preferable to the carbon copy look to which too many young people subscribe.

look like any one person, just types—like jocks or punks, or long hairs or normal."

In helping teens develop an individual look, explains Van Sickle, "We look at each person and say, 'What are the strong points of this person's face and what are the liabilities?' We try to help each person develop the best style with the least work—a look that won't take hours to perfect each morning." Key to that analysis, she adds, is the effort to convince teenage girls to use a minimal amount of makeup, an effort that teenage boys seem to applaud.

"High cheekbones and not too much makeup—that's how I like a girl to look," says Terry, 17.

Robert, 17, is more adamant about his aversion to excessive make-up: "If a girl wears a lot of makeup, then nine times out of ten she's real wild and thinks she's God's gift to men."

Mike, 15, agrees. "I just can't understand why some girls wear so much makeup. They don't even look real."

Finally, everyone agrees that regardless of whether facial features fit the classic mode or a more individualistic melting pot, the most important aspect of one's appearance is the personality that shines through. No one can make it today based solely on exterior beauty.

In fact, concludes Van Sickle, who often places models with top New York and European agencies, "Give me a mediocre-looking guy or girl with personality anytime over a screaming beauty with none. I can sign that person and she'll get work. Personality shows in a photograph, just as in real life."

II

*Looking Your Best
—Naturally*

3

A Healthful Lifestyle Enhances Natural Beauty

"Do candy and cokes and all that stuff really cause face problems?" asks Randy, 15, as he munches on a Mounds bar.

"My mom is always telling me to get off the couch and go get some fresh air," complains Jenny, 14. "Is she being just a little hyper or can exercise truly help my looks?"

"Now that my body isn't growing anymore, do I really still need eight hours of sleep every night to look good?" is 16-year-old Rebecca's question.

You've heard it more times than you want to: You are what you eat. It's just as true about other things you do for and to your body. Teens who eat sensibly, get enough sleep, and exercise regularly are healthier, feel fit, and exude a glow that makeup alone can't replace. Those are good habits to help you look great.

Moreover, teens who succumb to bad habits, such as smoking, drinking, and drug use, are going to see their lifestyles reflected on their faces. The difference is, that reflection won't be a pretty one.

Good Habits for Good Looks

Feed your face wisely—Generally the condition of your face, like the rest of your body, is reflected by a healthful diet. And while acne—a major problem for many teens—is not considered a dietary disease (see chapter 4), proper nutrition is indeed important for strong bones and teeth; a vibrant, taut complexion; bright eyes; and healthy, manageable hair. Moreover, good nutrition affects not just the part of your face that's visible but the underlying systems as well: the nerves, blood system, and underlying tissues.

Experts today advise a diet higher in fruits, vegetables (especially the leafy green ones), and complex carbohydrates—such as whole grains and pasta—and lower in fats and cholesterol. If you have a tendency to be overweight, watch calories. Eating a balanced diet will ensure that you receive the right proportion of vitamins and trace minerals without worrying about supplements.

How can you maintain good eating habits when everyone gathers at the closest pizza parlor or burger place? More and more fast food restaurants are offering salad bars; many have lowfat yogurt as well. Avoid french fries, cokes, and shakes when possible.

Finally, have something small with your friends and eat a more balanced meal at home. After all, it's the companionship and not the junk food that contributes to your good time. For more on what you should eat to maintain your good looks, check out the chart on the following page.

Eat Your Way to Good Looks

Your Problem	What You Need	Where to Get It
Acne, skin eruptions, blotchy complexion	Vitamin A Zinc Vitamins B-1, B-2, and B-6	Apricots, broccoli, milk, butter, spinach, tangerines. Liver, dark turkey meat, whole-grain breads, bran. Meat, fish, poultry, whole-grain breads and cereals, many fruits and vegetables.
Flabby skin	Silenium maintains the skin's elasticity; too much, though, can be toxic.	Poultry, seafood, red meat.
Pale complexion	Folic acid	Asparagus, broccoli, spinach, liver.
Bleeding gums	Vitamin C	Citrus fruits, cantaloupe, berries, tomatoes, broccoli.
Tooth decay	Calcium Vitamin D	Skim milk, cheese, yogurt. Fortified milk, liver, eggs, fish.
Dull, lifeless hair	Vitamin B-12	Lean meat, fish, eggs, milk, liver.
Premature hair loss	Zinc	Liver, dark turkey meat, whole-grain breads, bran.

Exercise often—Exercise has been called the world's most natural makeup, helping to give a healthy glow. This is because strenuous activity increases your blood's circulation to your face. Moreover, perspiration helps rid your complexion of oils and cellular waste products (the skin has been called the body's third kidney for this reason). Be sure to wash your face well after exercise, however (see chapter 4).

Exercise also is a great stress reducer. When your body gets moving, greater amounts of a hormone called beta-endorphin are produced. This reduces the appetite, improves your overall

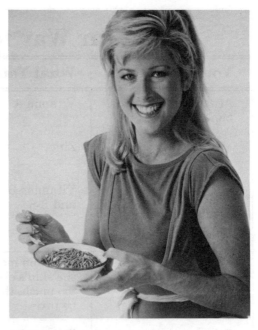

What you put into your body has a great deal to do with how good you look. Exercise helps, too.

mood, and reduces stress. Since stress has been linked to complexion problems, jogging it away makes sense. Better to take out your frustrations on a soccer ball than to let them show up in another pimple. Exercise gets your body systems working, especially your circulation. This sends a good supply of healthy, oxygenated blood through your body, cleansing out toxins and leaving skin with that glowing look. Consistent exercise also can control weight and reduce roundness or excessive fat in the facial area.

In short, couch potatoes soon end up looking pretty lumpy—facial features and all. If you absolutely must spend hours watching MTV, at least get up and dance to the music.

Get enough sleep—Fatigue is a common complaint of teenagers and one often caused simply by lack of sleep, although stress, depression, and lack of exercise also can be at fault. Teens have lots to do and often cut back severely on sleep, even though their bodies are still growing. In terms of your appearance, lack of sleep can affect your circulation, causing blood to be diverted from your face to major organs. Lack of sleep also contributes to dark circles and puffiness under your eyes.

Bad Habits to Avoid If You Value Your Appearance

"I know plenty of people who smoke, and they don't look any different to me," comments Susan, 14.

"I have a friend who does drugs," acknowledges Kathleen, 15. "I know they're not good for you, but I don't understand how they affect your face."

"Lots of kids drink," says Mark, 17. "They look okay to me."

There are all sorts of reasons to avoid smoking, drinking, and drugs—three life-threatening habits that adolescents are particularly susceptible to. One big reason is appearance. Just as with the foods you eat, the toxins that you take into your body eventually will show up on your face. Let's look at the damage they do.

Smoking:
* Constricts the small blood vessels of your face, reducing the supply of oxygen to delicate facial tissues. Eventually this will destroy that healthy glow that most teens admire, leaving you with a grayish "smoker's face."
* Contributes to lines around your face and eyes. Taking a drag on a cigarette causes your mouth to "purse up." While they may

not be noticeable in the teen years, eventually these lines around your mouth become permanent. Wrinkles around your eyes develop even sooner—experts aren't sure if this is the result of reduced oxygen to the face or because cigarette smoke causes squinting.

• Stains your teeth and spoils your smile. Smoking also is directly linked to mouth and throat cancers. Incidentally, the chewing tobacco popular today might not make your clothes smell bad, but it does stain your teeth and contribute to oral cancer.

Drugs:

• Cause acne flare-ups (especially "speed" or amphetamines).

• Suppress circulation to your skin, causing it to lose its natural color and look gray and tired. This is true of both stimulants and depressants, including the caffeine that is in colas, tea, and coffee.

• Contribute to nasal problems. This is a particular danger with cocaine, which can lead to nosebleeds and breathing difficulties, destroy the cartilage within your nose, and even cause your entire nose to collapse.

• Cause facial lines and wrinkles. This is as true of marijuana as it is of conventional cigarettes.

• Cause fluid retention that results in a roundness or distortion of your face if the drugs are steroids or synthetic male hormones.

Drinking:

• Dehydrates your skin by drawing water away from its surface. Healthy skin needs this moisture.

• Increases the problem of broken capillaries.

• Causes blood vessels to expand, or dilate, increasing the redness of your skin. An alcohol "glow" is too red to look healthy.

• Lowers your physical reaction time, thus contributing to accidents, especially those involving motorcycles and automobiles. The facial damage from such accidents is a leading cause of facial disfigurement for teens (see chapter 12).

4

How to Get and Keep a Glowing Complexion

"My face is in perfect shape except for my blemishes," comments Amy, 14, speaking for many teens across the country. "I'd do anything to get rid of them."

Dan, 16, asks with an air of resignation, "Is there anything that truly will get rid of acne? I've tried everything you can buy, and nothing works."

"Kids who have bad acne sometimes have a hard time getting dates at our school," remarks Justin, 16.

A clear complexion is the number one concern of teenagers across the country. With a little effort, it's a goal that most can achieve.

First of all, know that if you have acne, you are not alone. The National Center for Health Statistics reports that of American adolescents between the ages of 12 and 17, fewer than 30 percent have naturally clear skin.

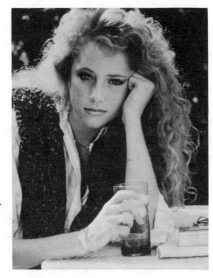

A beautifully clear complexion is the desire of every teenager.

Acne is genetically flawed skin—it does not have the ability to keep itself clean. Moreover, adolescence is a time when hormonal changes intensify your skin's tendency to erupt. While acne is an inherited problem, and a lifelong one as well, the changes of puberty aggravate the situation. Moreover, since your appearance is deemed so important during teen years, an outbreak of acne can cause internal anguish—stress, in simpler terms—that leads, in a frustrating cycle, to a worsening of the acne.

"I can't believe it!" wails Suzanne, 15. "My face was fine for weeks and now that the prom is just two days away, I have enormous zits. Why is this happening to me?"

David, 16, points out that his complexion was fine all summer long but now it has broken out. "Is my skin allergic to school, too?"

Dermatologists report they often see more teenagers for complexion problems just as the school year is to begin. Going back to school, with all its social undercurrents, can be quite stressful. The relationship between stress and acne also explains why your face has a maddening habit of breaking out just before a very important date or that book report you have to give in front of your whole class.

You may wonder how teen acne gets started. The change in hormonal level during adolescence causes your *sebaceous glands* (the oil glands of your face and other parts of your body) to overproduce. The result may be simply an oily complexion. The excess oil, however, also may clog the opening of the pores and cause blackheads. If these are not removed, bacteria may build up within the pore duct, and infection can cause pimples. In more serious cases, cysts can result.

The good news is that acne can be controlled. There are various courses of treatment available, some requiring the supervision of a physician, and not all will work for everyone. Basically, acne treatments fall into three categories: topical preparations, oral medications, and specialized treatments. We'll look at each in turn, but first, let's consider cleanliness.

Keeping your face scrupulously clean is most important. You may not be able to stop the oil from being produced, but you can remove it from your face frequently. Use a good cleanser, not a harsh soap. There are special soaps with mild abrasives in them that can be helpful. Neutrogena® acne soap and Acnaveen, which contains oatmeal, are two that work for many teens. Use of an astringent after cleansing your face is helpful. Keeping your hair clean and off your face will help keep oil under control as well.

Topical Preparations for Treating Acne

• Nonprescription creams, lotions, and gels. You can buy these almost anywhere skincare products are sold. They dry the skin and work for mild acne cases. Many of these contain benzoyl peroxide in a 2.5, 5, or 10 percent solution that helps kill surface bacteria.

• Topical antibiotics. These often come packaged in an alcohol lotion or gel form. They, too, dry the skin and fight bacteria.

Is Retin-A® for You?

Retin-A® has been called the miracle cream for its newly discovered ability to smooth wrinkles. But for years its primary use has been for a skin condition of far more interest to teens than wrinkles: acne. It does work, everyone agrees, but this is not an over-the-counter preparation and must be used under the supervision of a physician. Different skin types react to Retin-A® in very differing ways. Fair-skinned, blue-eyed teens, for example, are likely to experience far more drying and scaling of the face than those with darker hair and complexions.

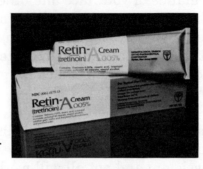

Any cream is a miracle if it clears the complexion.

Retin-A® increases the sensitivity of the skin to the sun's ultraviolet rays and always should be used with a sunblock of at least 15. The cream actually thins the skin's outer, dead layer, making it far more susceptible to serious sun damage. Thus, it makes sense not to start on a Retin-A® regimen just before a skiing trip or a vacation at the beach.

Your physician will monitor your dosage. For some people, a mere dab is plenty. For others, more is better. Most users will want to follow application of the cream with a moisturizer to counteract the dryness it causes. Physicians say lower concentrations are likely in the near future, making Retin-A® easier to use. Experts say daily use for two to three months is necessary until improvement is first noticed; longer use is preferable.

• Retin-A®. A relatively new product (since the seventies) available only by prescription (consult your family doctor or a dermatologist), Retin-A® is a derivative of vitamin A, known generically as tretinoin, that comes in a cream or gel for application to the face. (See opposite page for more on this popular new cream.)

Oral Medications for Treating Acne

• Oral antibiotics. Tetracycline and erythromycin are antibiotics often prescribed for moderate to severe acne. The purpose is to reduce the bacteria that collect in the pores. Sometimes dosages have to be adjusted for best results. Generally the antibiotic is taken daily in pill form. Antibiotics should only be taken under the direction of a physician.

• Accutane®. Also taken in pill form, Accutane® is a much more aggressive treatment for acne. A derivative of vitamin A, Accutane® has come under heavy attack because of its connection to birth defects. Any girl who is pregnant should not take Accutane®. For severe acne, Accutane® often is amazingly effective. It is taken daily for a period of five months and then discontinued. (Because of the extreme side effects, other dosages are sometimes used. Accutane® requires medical supervision.) Following the course of treatment, the acne often disappears altogether, although it may recur after a period of several years, requiring a second course of Accutane® treatment.

There are various side effects associated with Accutane®, among them extreme dryness of the lips and mucous membranes. The lips often crack and peel, and exposure to the sun should be avoided. Other occasionally seen side effects include headaches and muscle and joint pain.

Specialized Acne Treatments

• Comedone extraction. The comedo extractor is a small appliance that can be placed directly over a blackhead (also known as a *comedo*) and used to extract it. It will not cause scarring. The extractor is available from a physician or pharmacy; teens can use it at home, thus reducing office visits. One caution: The extractor should not be used on pimples, which are infected blackheads, since the pressure at that stage can damage the surrounding skin.

• Liquid nitrogen. This is a spray that reduces acne's inflammation and lightly peels the skin to open clogged pores. The procedure is performed in a dermatologist's office.

 by Cathy Guisewite

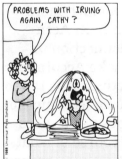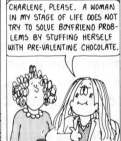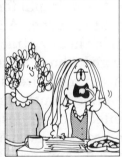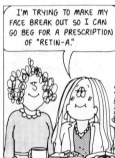

• Ultraviolet light. Used in very small dosages—just minutes—ultraviolet light works like sunlight to dry the skin. Because of the danger of ultraviolet rays, consider this option only at the suggestion of a physician.

• Intralesional steroids. Mild steroids can at times be injected into acne cysts to reduce inflammation and pain.

For teens whose acne lesions already have resulted in scarring, see chapter 9 for facial plastic surgery treatments to minimize the scars.

Of Sweat, Shaving, Chocolate, and Those Frustrating Zits

"Are candy, cokes, and all that fast food really the cause of my face breaking out?" asks Peggy, who's convinced her diet causes pimples.
While some teens do seem to notice an increase in skin eruptions when they eat certain foods, such as chocolate, salted nuts, or greasy french fries, medical science has not been able to draw a conclusive link between diet and acne in everyone. However, if a particular food makes your skin problems worse, avoid eating it as much as possible.

Janice, 13, has an interesting concern. "Can sleeping on the same pillowcase for a long time cause your cheeks to break out?"
Perhaps. Teen skin tends to be oily and attracts dirt and bacteria. If you work hard during the day at keeping your face clean and free of oil, it doesn't make much sense to sleep on a pillowcase that has not been laundered recently.

"Does being active in sports cause acne?" asks Joel, 17.
Being active in sports does not cause acne. An exception is when equipment is worn that rubs an area prone to problems, such as a

The Dangers of a Beautiful Tan

"How tan you are is a big deal," explains Lucy, 17. "I have a good figure, but I hate to be seen in a bathing suit because I'm so pale."

"Girls look great with a tan," says beach aficionado Robin, 15. "But when they burn instead of tan, it looks stupid."

"I never burn," declares olive-skinned Naomi, 13. "Does this mean I'm not damaging my skin like some of my friends who do burn?"

Most teens agree: A great-looking tan is a must in the summertime. But while the effects of the sun's rays may be a boon to your social life, they're downright damaging to your skin. Actually, it's the ultraviolet rays that do the damage. There are two kinds: *UVA* and *UVB*. UVA rays are longer, act more slowly, but penetrate more deeply into your skin. They are of equal intensity all day long and throughout the year, so they can damage your skin in winter as well as in the early morning or late afternoon. UVB rays are shorter, have greater intensity in the summer and midday hours, and will quickly burn your skin.

Tanning booths are particularly damaging. In fact, today's tanning booths, which use the slower UVA radiation, may actually cause more long-term damage than the old UVB booths. Although the newer booths do not produce a noticeable burn as quickly as the old ones, the deeper penetration of UVA rays means more serious long-term effects, such as skin cancer.

Melanin, a brownish pigment that determines skin color, provides natural protection from the sun. Naomi is right: People with dark or olive skin do seem to have more natural protection from the damaging ultraviolet rays.

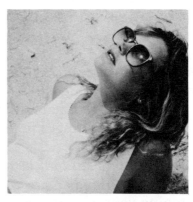

Acquiring a deep, bronzed tan each summer is a major goal of both guys and girls. Magazine swimsuit beauties are never shown with pale skin, furthering the popularity of the tanned look. But too much sun can be decidedly unhealthful, physicians now say.

Of course, it is unrealistic to suggest that no one get a summer tan. For the safest tan, the American Medical Association recommends a sunscreen with an SPF (sun protection factor) of at least 15 applied every 40 to 60 minutes. If you have freckles, use SPF 28 or 29 to block their spread. It is important to know that sunscreen must be absorbed into the skin in order to be effective. Thus, it should be applied from a half-hour to two full hours before going out into the sun. Dermatologists tell us that the most effective use of a sunscreen is daily and year-round—some moisturizers include sunscreen protection. If your skin is oily, choose a drying, gel-type sunscreen. For dry skin, use a liquid formula. A sun visor or hat also will protect your face while sunbathing, participating in sports, and doing yard work. Protecting lips and the area around your eyes is particularly important.

A final note: Those beauties modeling swimwear may look tan, but don't think for a minute that they're letting the sun ruin their skin. Those tans are all bronze makeup gel, a not-well-kept modeling industry secret.

headband for tennis. Perspiration that dries on your skin acts as an irritant, so clean your face carefully after any strenuous activity.

"Why does my face always break out before my period?" laments Maria, 17. "I feel bad enough without my face being a mess, too."
Your hormones fluctuate dramatically just before the onset of your period, causing changes in the level of oil production then.

Paul, 18, points out that he has trouble shaving because of his acne. "Is there anything to make this easier?"
Softening your whiskers with soap and warm water before shaving will help. Use a sharp blade and try to avoid nicking the blemishes, which causes them to bleed.

"I know the sun is supposed to be bad for the skin, but it seems to clear up my acne," points out Jon, 17.
He's right. In a dry climate, controlled sun exposure—with a proper sunscreen—will help dry an acne problem. A humid climate tends to increase oil production.

"I get hairspray build-up along my bangs," notes Sharon, 17. "It makes the skin on my upper forehead break out. What can I do?"
When applying hairspray, shield your face with your hand, then use an astringent to clean your face. Finally, when your mother nags at you for picking at your face, listen up. Using your fingers to push out blackheads or open pimples can damage the tissues and increase the possibility of scarring. Your fingers also leave bacteria. If you have a pimple that is really driving you crazy, apply a warm, moist washcloth to it. Wrap your fingers in a tissue and apply gentle pressure to the area. This may do the trick. Do not force it, however, and be sure to cleanse your face well afterward.

5

Facial Sculpting with Cosmetics

"I know a girl whose makeup is always perfect," notes Maria, 14. "She knows exactly what to use to bring out the best features of her face. Any advice for the rest of us?"

"When I look at makeovers in the magazines, I'm amazed sometimes at how they can get rid of blotchy skin and make nondescript eyes look great and even make a big nose or wide chin seem to disappear," comments Sharon, 16. "I never seem to get the same effect."

Your face may be of classic proportions or reflect great individual style. Nonetheless, you still may have facial features that would look better if they weren't so prominent or features that would be more striking with just a little accentuation.

With the proper techniques at your fingertips, you can indulge in *facial sculpting*: the art of using makeup subtly to call attention to your best features and disguise the rest. There are three steps to this process. First, prepare your skin with foundation to even its tone, eliminate blotchiness, and cover minor imperfections; then use cosmetics to enhance facial features; finally, choose a hairstyle that complements your facial shape and profile.

Setting the Foundation
"The purpose of makeup is to define features and even out skin tones," says Diane Young, a corrective skin counselor in New York City. Foundation should match the skin tone as closely as possible and should be used only to even out the color, not as a mask. If the skin is in good condition, some pressed translucent powder is fine.

For skin that is particularly blotchy in appearance, an underbase skin toner may be necessary. Toners, available in green, yellow, and purple, go on under the foundation to neutralize skin discolorations. A green underbase is recommended for the excessive redness teen skin often presents. If you do have a reddened complexion, avoid makeup colors like rose, red, or hot pink. Soft shades of green and blue in your makeup and clothing will neutralize the redness. For evening out the lack of pigmentation on certain parts of the face, commonly around the mouth and eyes, that is caused by a condition known as true *vitiligo*, try a quick tanning substance as a camouflage. A drug known as Psoralnes can be taken internally or used directly on the skin to make it more sensistive to the sun. This allows the user to get a low-grade sunburn that sometimes causes the melanin to return.

"Does makeup make your complexion worse?" asks Judy, 13, who has just received permission to start wearing cosmetics.

According to Young, makeup will not clog your pores or make your complexion worse if you follow these two steps: Use the moisturizer recommended for your skin type, and cleanse your face thoroughly before going to bed. If breakouts are a problem, use water-based, oil-free, noncomedogenic (will not clog pores) cosmetics. There are inexpensive products available in all cosmetic lines.

Using Makeup to Your Best Advantage

The basic trick to remember in facial sculpting is that dark colors make features appear to recede while lighter colors make them appear more prominent. Use this principle in accentuating your own best features.

"All of the models seem to have beautiful, high cheekbones. How can I get that look?"

To create the illusion of high cheekbones, draw dots of highlighter (foundation or coverstick a couple of shades lighter than you normally use) from the top of each cheekbone to your hairline. Blend. Then take a darker shade of coverstick or powder and make a similar line under the bottom edge of each cheekbone. Blend with a damp sponge and apply blush as usual.

Incidentally, says Young, a little blush goes a long way. You're

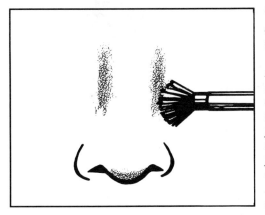

"My nose is really too wide for the rest of my face. Is there any way to make it look smaller?"

For a thinner-looking nose, draw a line with light coverstick down the center of your nose. Gently blend with your fingertip. Next, draw a parallel line on either side of your nose with a darker shade of pressed powder or coverstick. Blend, preferably with a sponge, to soften the effect. If your nose is still a problem, see chapter 6.

trying to enhance, not cover. Applying blush just along your cheek-bone is out, but don't extend your blush below the hollow part of your cheek. Applying a touch of blush lightly on your forehead and chin will balance the effect. (Some models have cheek implants inserted, something not recommended for teens. See chapter 11.)

"Is there any way to cover freckles completely?"

There are a number of good cosmetics available for concealment that were developed originally for covering up freckles. For freckles, moles, minor scars, and other blemishes, try Dermablend or Covermark. Most drugstores carry them. For large, disfiguring scars, birthmarks, and blemishes that cannot be covered with makeup, see chapter 9.

"Everyone comments about large, deep-set eyes—they're so romantic. How can I use eye makeup to my best advantage?"

The eyes, indeed, are the facial features girls most like to highlight. You can create many different effects using makeup around your eyes. First, study the proportions of the ideal eye and eyebrow in figure 4 at right, then try to achieve that effect with makeup. Note in the drawing the angle at which the brow arches above the eye and the angle of the eye in proportion to the outer edge of the nose. To highlight your eyes and minimize their defects, first apply highlighter to the area between

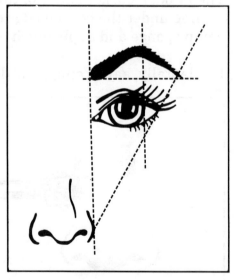

Figure 4

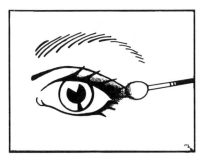

Applying a slightly darker shade of eyeshadow to the outer corners of your eyes will make them seem wider apart.

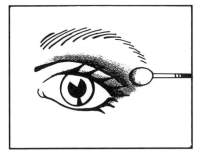

A darker shadow applied to your brow bone will make the area seem to recede, something a pastel cannot accomplish.

your lashes and brow. Then try the following effects if your eyes need to be:

• *Larger*—brush shadow out to the sides along your orbital bone (the bone that forms the eye socket). Lighter colors give the illusion that the area is larger. Extra eye liner in the outer corners gives the illusion of opening and widening. White or bone soft pencil on your lid's inner portion also creates a more wide-eyed effect.

• *More prominent*—apply shadow above your lid and extend it toward your brow. Use a different, lighter shade on your lid. Blue, sable, or teal shades of pencil applied to the lower inner portion of your lid make the white of your eye appear whiter.

• *Less drooping*—brush color upward at the outer corner of your eye. Use a second, lighter color to blend in at your orbital bone.

• *Less hooded*—use darker shades of shadow to make the hooded area appear to recede. Eyeliner should be more intense along your upper lashline.

Asian eyes, which have no lid crease and very little lid showing, need a heavier application of eyeliner to the upper lashline for dimension. With eye shadow, use lighter shades to diminish the impact of a fleshy or prominent brow bone.

For bags and dark circles under your eyes, the same coverstick used for blemishes and blotchy skin should work. Blend it gently so as not to damage delicate tissues around your eyes. For more serious eye problems, such as lids that droop so much they interfere with your vision, see chapter 8.

Applied correctly, makeup can conceal a number of facial problems. Sometimes, however, it isn't easy to achieve the results you need. To learn correct makeup application techniques, Young recommends that teens take a lesson from a professional. "There is a lot of free advice available, in addition to books and magazines," she states. Beauty schools and salons often give free makeover demonstrations. There are demonstrations and cosmetologists, very willing to give free advice, at cosmetic counters in large department stores. Your local paper may announce special programs. If there is a fee, it is usually minimal and often can be applied against purchase of a particular line of cosmetics.

Make Sure Your Hair and Face Work Together

"I think hair is the only way guys can express themselves, facially," says Mike, 18. *"It's important, though, that your hair look styled."*

"Even if you aren't great looking, you can look good by curling your hair or moussing it and always taking care of it," adds Megan, 16.

Kathleen, 15, adds, "My head was sort of a strange shape when I was a kid, so my mother let my hair grow long and thick to conceal it. People saw my hair and never noticed the shape of my head."

Just as cosmetics can help bring out your best facial features, so can the proper hairstyle help put your face in balance. Determine your face shape and the best hairstyle (see page 50 for suggestions), and then ask your stylist to design a style for you as close to that ideal as your particular hair will allow. Obviously a straight style with thick bangs won't work if your hair is kinky and uncontrollable. A good stylist, however, can suggest an alternate style.

It's possible that even the artful use of makeup and hairstyle won't solve your particular facial problem. If the problem is serious enough to cause you considerable anguish on a daily basis — especially if you find it difficult to focus on other aspects of your life — the upcoming sections will provide the information you need to consider another possible option: facial plastic surgery. As you consider this option, bear in mind that facial plastic surgery, as any surgery, is a serious and often irrevocable undertaking that should not be entered into lightly. Moreover, your parents should be involved in every step of the decision-making process.

MISS PEACH MELL LAZARUS

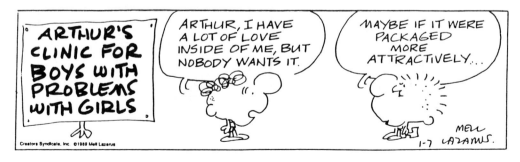

Consider Your Profile
When Choosing a Hairstyle

There are three basic profiles to consider when choosing the best hairstyle: straight, concave, and convex. The proper hairstyle can help your profile appear straight—the ideal shape. Such deception also helps to minimize prominent features, such as a large nose or an extended chin.

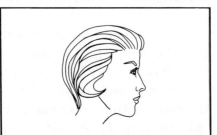 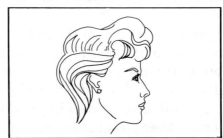

STRAIGHT

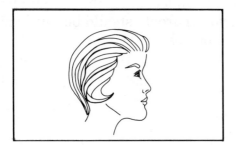 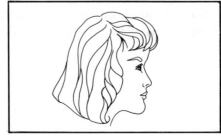

CONCAVE

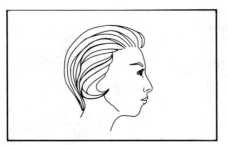 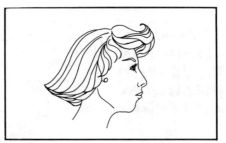

CONVEX

III

Facial Plastic Surgery Is an Option . . .

6

. . . If Your Nose Doesn't Fit Your Face

"I absolutely hate my nose," declares Mary Beth, 18, in a familiar complaint. "It doesn't stick out, but it's very wide on the sides when I smile, and I get very self-conscious about it."

"I know a girl at school who would be very pretty if it weren't for the fact that she has a very big nose," offers Jennifer, 17.

Melissa, 15, adds that a guy at her school has an obvious hook nose. "Everyone calls him 'Toucan.'"

Have you ever wished that you could "do something" about your nose? If your nose truly is unattractive—and your problem cannot be solved by changing your hairstyle or by the artful use of cosmetics—facial plastic surgery may offer you an alternative.

Certain features of your nose can be reshaped or refined. If your nose has a hump on top; if it has been broken; if it projects outward too far; if it is crooked, too long, too wide, or too big for your face; if the tip of your nose is big and bulbous, or if it points downward like a hawk's bill—your appearance may be changed through a type of surgery called *rhinoplasty*. A rhinoplasty can help to refine your nose and bring it in line with your other facial features.

Again, facial plastic surgery is not for everyone. The results are not reversible, and no surgeon can guarantee that you will be happy with the results. Also, every surgical procedure has its risks.

Some Common Concerns and Questions

"How is nose surgery done?" "Is it done internally?" "Are there any scars?"

Usually the incisions used in nose surgery are hidden just inside the rim of the nostrils. Sometimes, though, skin incisions are also needed. When used, they are placed on the bottom of the nose and are easily hidden in the natural creases where your nose meets your cheeks and lip. For example, to make flaring nostrils smaller, the surgeon may make an incision at the bottom edge of each nostril. In some cases, it may also be necessary to make a small, inconspicuous incision between the nostrils.

"I don't understand how a surgeon can possibly reconstruct the bone of the nose to make it look good."

"I've heard they have to break the nose first. Is this true?"

Many people having nose surgery worry that the doctor is going to break their nose. This is one of the big myths of nose surgery. Actually, the doctor carves the bone or shaves a little of it away in order to change the shape of the nose. By adjusting the shape of the underlying bone and removing excess cartilage and bone, the surgeon can make the nose more narrow or less crooked, remove a hump, or downturn a pug nose. Then the structures of the nose are carefully repositioned, an outside splint is applied to hold them in place, and the skin is allowed to heal to the new framework.

"Where is the surgery done?"

Some facial plastic surgeons have surgical suites right in their office. Others use ambulatory care facilities (where one-day surgery is performed) or the outpatient departments of local hospitals. The surgery can be performed comfortably and safely using a combination of intravenous sedation and local anesthesia so you can recover quickly. If you need extensive surgery, or if you are especially nervous, your surgeon may advise general anesthesia so that you are completely asleep.

"Does nose surgery hurt?"

Your surgeon will do everything possible to make you comfortable. Pain is minimal during the operation, and you may not even remember anything of the surgery afterward. The procedure takes about one to two hours, depending on how much work must be done.

"What does your face look like after the surgery?"

Immediately after surgery, you will find yourself wearing a small splint or cast on your nose. This usually stays on for five to seven days after surgery. You will have some temporary swelling around your nose and some bruising at the inner corners of your eyes and on your lower eyelids, a normal result of surgery. The bruising subsides in a few days to several weeks, and most of the swelling disappears within a few months. It can take six months to a year for the swelling to disappear entirely. Your nose will look better immediately, but you won't see the "finished product" for up to a year. After two weeks, however, your nose will be "socially acceptable."

"Doesn't facial plastic surgery on your nose make breathing hard?"

Your nose will probably feel stuffy after surgery because there is usually some internal swelling and nasal packing. Your doctor may give you a medication to reduce the swelling and ease the stuffiness, which generally lasts between one and three weeks. You should notice a big improvement when the splint is removed, and your breathing will improve as the swelling continues to go down.

"Do you have to breathe through your mouth the whole time healing is taking place?"

You should be able to breathe through your nose within a day or two, particularly if you follow your doctor's instructions carefully. Some surgeons use a light internal dressing inside the nostrils. If this is used, you will have to breathe through your mouth until it is removed, which varies between one day and one week.

"Does nose surgery have any long-term effects on your breathing?"

Many people find that they actually breathe better after surgery. Cosmetic surgery on the nose does not involve the area where the air goes through, but your facial plastic surgeon will examine your airway, and if it needs improvement, he can work on it at the same time. Some people don't even realize that their breathing is not as good as it could be, and are pleasantly surprised to find that they can breathe much better after their nose surgery.

"Can nose surgery correct breathing problems?"

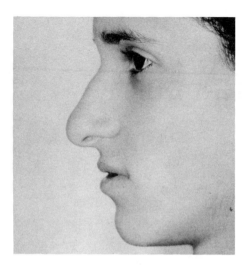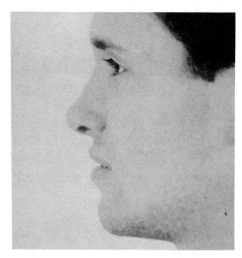

This young man had to have two rhinoplasty procedures for the facial plastic surgeon to remove the necessary cartilage (before, at left) to get the desired result (at right).

If you have problems caused by physical obstructions in your nose —difficult breathing, chronic sinus problems, recurring headaches, and the like—you may need an operation called *septorhinoplasty*. This procedure improves blockages in your nasal passages through incisions placed inside your nose. If you have a cosmetic problem, the exterior of your nose can be corrected at the same time.

"Will having nose surgery affect the sound of my voice?"

Not unless you had severe obstructions inside your nose to begin with. Some people with serious blockages to the breathing passages may have a voice that is very nasal. When surgery is done to correct the breathing problems, the voice usually loses its nasal tone and becomes more normal. Most people having nose surgery will not notice any change in the sound of their voice.

Nebraska Teen Gets Nose Surgery for Her Birthday

Two years ago, Jennifer of Nebraska received what she considers one of the best birthday presents ever: nose surgery.

"I was almost 16 when I had the surgery," she explains. "In fact, the bandages came off on my birthday. What a present that was! I could tell the improvement right away. My face was a little swollen, but it wasn't all that noticeable. I had just a little bruising, a few smudges under my eyes that I could easily cover with makeup."

Like many teens, Jennifer didn't hate her nose, exactly, but she didn't like it much, either. "With a big hump and a down-turned tip, my nose certainly wasn't my best feature," she points out.

She remembers when she was little, her nose bothered her a lot. "Kids made fun of it sometimes.

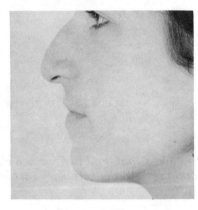

Jennifer before her nose surgery. . .

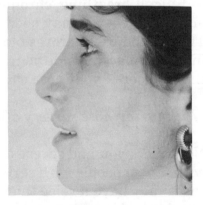

. . . and after surgery was completed just before her 16th birthday.

But I never really had problems making friends. Eventually I learned to joke about it and just laugh off the comments. I knew that none of my friends really meant to be mean."

When Jennifer was in her mid-teens, her parents mentioned the possibility of a rhinoplasty. "They didn't pressure me or anything," she's quick to point out. "They just let me know that they would go along with it if I ever wanted to get something done about my nose. I had never thought about nose surgery as a real possibility before. But once the idea was out in the open, I started thinking seriously about it."

The operation went so smoothly and painlessly that Jennifer doesn't even remember it. She explains, "I took these pills, and they put an intravenous line in my arm. The next thing I knew I was in the recovery room with a bandage on my face, and my parents were there. I know some kids have pain with this type of surgery, but for me it was not painful at all. I never even took a pain killer."

She continues: "I took it easy for about a week while the bandage was on, but friends would come over and we'd go out for ice cream, stuff like that. The bandage didn't bother me too much."

Having a new nose, says Jennifer, didn't change her life dramatically. "I've always been an outgoing person," she says, "so that didn't change. It was more of a gradual thing. In some ways, I think having a big nose when I was young helped me become a stronger person. I have more confidence. And I really like what I see when I look in the mirror."

"Can nasal damage caused by drug abuse be corrected with this type of nose surgery?"

Drug abuse can cause perforations (holes) in the nasal septum (the internal wall of the nose). This type of damage can sometimes be repaired by surgery, but such repair surgery is not always successful. In fact, really large perforations may be irreparable because of the danger that surgery will collapse the nose. The most important steps are to stop using the drugs that caused the problem and to seek advice.

"What are the risks of this surgery?"

Every surgical procedure involves risks. However, cosmetic nose surgery carries a much lower risk of complications than many other forms of surgery. Your facial plastic surgeon will tell you about the risks of nose surgery at your first appointment. For instance, there is a small chance of bleeding, which may require nasal packing. In a small percentage of cases, infection may set in and require treatment. Occasionally, a touch-up procedure may be needed in six months or a year.

Making the Decision

How do you make the decision to have surgery on a problem nose? There are many things to consider. Not everyone with a big or a crooked nose will want to have surgery. Lots of people have become successful, even famous—in spite of a big nose.

Susan, 16, points out that she knows a girl with a real big nose, "but it really doesn't bother her. She is outgoing and a nice person."

Jason, 16, thinks noses are overstated. "People in my school with big noses aren't made fun of, and they get dates, too."

Not everyone is bothered by an unusual facial feature. It's important to think about how you feel. If your nose really makes you unhappy, the decision to have it operated on rests with you. The best reason for getting a nose job is that you want to look better and feel better about yourself. You should never have your nose or any other facial feature reshaped to please someone else—even your parents—if you, yourself, are happy with it as it is.

Will having the size or shape of your nose surgically changed help you get dates? Don't count on it. If you are counting on surgery to improve your social life, you probably shouldn't have the operation. Facial plastic surgery promises to improve your outward appearance, nothing more. What's on the inside is up to you!

"I have a really terrible-looking nose," explains Brad, 16. "I wonder how much a nose can be changed?"

That really depends on what your nose looks like and how much change you feel you need. If you have a big problem—say, a huge nose that overpowers your face—you may need more correction to get the improvement you want than would someone with just a tiny hump. Even if you do opt for a major change, and you have successful surgery, you may be surprised to find that many of your friends won't even notice the difference. There are limits to what facial plastic surgery can accomplish, and you should be sure you understand those limits. Your expectations have to be reasonable.

Ann, 13, wants to know, "How much does surgery on your nose change your whole facial appearance?"

Again, that depends. Successful nose surgery may make a dramatic change in the rest of your face, because your nose is no longer drawing attention away from other attractive features. With your facial features in better balance, people may be more likely to notice features like your hair, your complexion, or your eyes. If having the surgery gives you a great psychological boost, it may even have a positive effect on your facial expression—you may relax and smile more because you feel so much better about yourself. On the other hand, don't expect surgery on your nose to improve the looks of your entire face. Remember, your nose is only one small part of your face, and it's important not to expect too much.

"I broke my nose five times," reveals Stephanie, 15. "Is there hope?"

There is always hope that a badly damaged nose can be improved. The facial plastic surgeon takes the same approach with a nose that has been broken as with any other problem nose: first deciding what is wrong with the way the nose looks and works, and then planning how surgery may improve the problems. Generally speaking, crooked noses can be straightened, humps can be removed, a wide nose can be narrowed, and a flat nose can be built up. If your nose has been damaged, discuss your concerns with a facial plastic surgeon you trust.

For Better or For Worse®   **by Lynn Johnston**

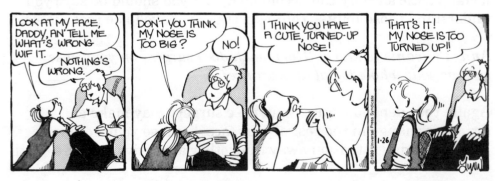

Planning the Surgery

You and your surgeon will work together to plan your surgery before the first incision is made. Your surgeon will probably take a number of photographs from several angles. This helps him or her to evaluate your problem and plan the procedure.

"But can you choose the nose you want?" asks Greg, 14.

Not exactly. Planning your surgery is not like going to the department store and picking out a new nose. The final result depends on what the surgeon has to work with. The goal of surgery is to improve upon what nature has provided, not to give you a new nose.

"Can the surgeon tell you what your nose will look like after surgery?" is the question that Charlie, 15, and many others have asked.

Your surgeon will spend a lot of time discussing what you want and helping you to visualize how surgery can improve the way your nose looks. Facial plastic surgeons have a variety of ways to show you what to expect. One doctor may point out possible changes in the mirror; another may prefer to sketch your profile and then draw how you might look with a different nose. Some take pictures and draw right on the photographs, or use plastic overlays to demonstrate the suggested changes.

The newest method, *computer-assisted imaging*, uses a video camera to put your face on a television screen and a computer pen to actually change the picture. Remember, though, the machine cannot predict exact surgical results. No surgeon can guarantee how you will look because every nose is different. Final results will depend on the extent of your problem, your age, ethnic background, skin type, and other facial features.

Sometimes Mother Does Know Best

Robin invested a lot of trust in her mother when she agreed to have her nose done six years ago at the age of 13.

"I was in the eighth grade," she explains, "and I had never heard of a rhinoplasty. My mother has a perfect little nose, but I had this wide thing with a bridge the width of my nostrils. It's amazing I didn't have a complex. My mother's suggestion was very perceptive. She knew eventually I would have problems about my nose."

When she went for the consultation, Robin recalls that the facial plastic surgeon took cotton swabs and covered up parts of her nose. "I looked in the mirror, and I was amazed at the difference. In this case Mommy certainly knew best."

And once the surgery was done? "Everyone just loved my nose. It's the most natural nose I've ever seen."

"I was overweight and having trouble in school socially," Robin, now a student at a Boston university, relates. "I was really a target for the other kids and had only one good friend. There was another girl at school who didn't like me, and she had an ugly nose, too. I used to joke that if I ever had a nose job, the two of us ought to have it together. Well, on the first day back to school after I had my rhinoplasty, this girl commented to someone else about me, 'I really hate Robin, but I have to admit her nose looks good.' If she was able to say that, I figured my nose looked really good, just exceptional."

Like all good facial plastic surgery, Robin's rhinoplasty was not a drastic change that made people's heads turn. "Something looked really good about me, but you couldn't tell what it was," she explains. "I went to visit my relatives in Israel, and they knew I looked good but had no idea why. It was only when we started looking at baby pictures that they figured it out. I didn't have that big wide nose anymore."

"Having nose surgery didn't turn my life around," she continues, "but it made me feel so much better about myself and that's what changed my life. I think the first thing you notice is someone's face. After I had my nose done, my eyes became huge. They're my best feature—even more than my perfect nose—but they weren't noticeable before." Having the surgery done early was important, Robin feels. "I didn't have a chance to get a complex. I feel like I was born with this nose—I hardly remember the other one."

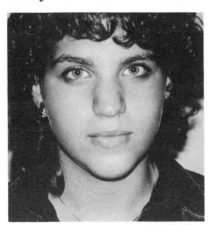 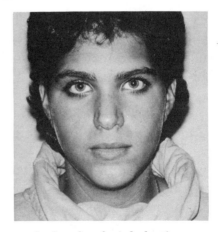

Robin's nose (before, at left) was improved when her facial plastic surgeon raised the tip and narrowed the width using soft tissue excision.

*"How old do I need to be to have facial plastic surgery on my nose?"
is 16-year-old Rachel's question.*

Much depends on your physical size and whether you are close to
reaching your maximum growth and facial development. Girls
need to be at least 13, boys about 15. Most young people who have
nose surgery are between 16 and 18.

After the Surgery

Once you decide to go through with surgery, you may wonder what
to expect afterward. You will be relieved to know that noses heal
quickly, and most people who have had the surgery report little or
no pain. There are other post-operative considerations, such as:

*"How soon will I be able to go back to my regular activities," asks
Jeremy, 16, a dedicated tennis player.*

You can return to school or work as soon as the splint is removed,
usually a week after surgery. You should avoid strenuous physical
activity for the first few weeks, but you will be able to do almost
anything after a month. Stay away from rugged contact sports for
six weeks, and protect your nose from the sun for about three
months, so that you do not get a burn that can cause your nose to
swell.

"Can I wear glasses or contacts after nose surgery?" asks Amy, 16.

Today's contact lenses can be worn as soon as you feel like it after
surgery. If you wear glasses, do not place them directly on your
nose for a month after surgery. Your doctor may give you a small
splint to keep them from putting pressure on your nose, or you can
suspend them from your forehead with a bit of tape.

7

...If Your Chin Is Weak or Your Mouth Is Small

"A girl at my school has a very weak chin and a huge nose—it makes her look as if she's about to bite me," comments Tim, 16.

"I hate my lips," declares Cassie, 15. "They are really thin and small. You can barely notice they're there."

"When I smile my gums show," notes Tess, 17. "I hate to smile because of it. Is there anything that can be done?"

Some problems are easily solved with careful use of cosmetics. Others are not so easy to disguise. Often, problems with the lower part of the face are in this category. If you have a weak chin, or if your chin is way too long; if your teeth don't fit together right, or your smile is "gummy"; if your lips are huge, or if they are barely there; if your lower face just seems out of proportion—you may want to consider facial plastic surgery to improve your appearance.

When the Problem Is Structural: Orthognathic Surgery

Problems with the lower face are often more than just cosmetic problems. If your jaws and teeth don't fit together properly, it can have a negative effect on both your appearance and your health. Structural problems like these can cause dental problems if they are not treated.

"Do they have to move bones around to fix a receding chin?" asks Jason, 19, with some trepidation.

Not always. It depends on what causes the receding chin. There are two main types of problems: Some people simply have a small chin and are best helped by chin implant surgery. Others may have

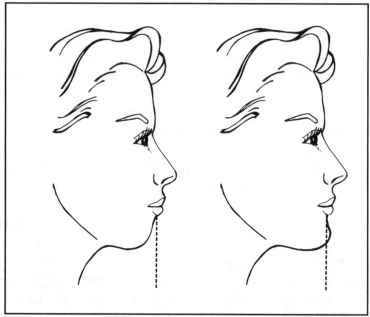

From the lower lip, a line extended straight down will fall in front of a receding chin, but cut through a protruding chin.

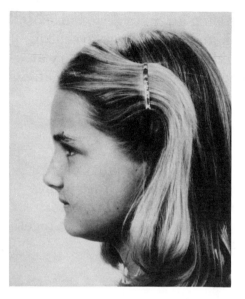 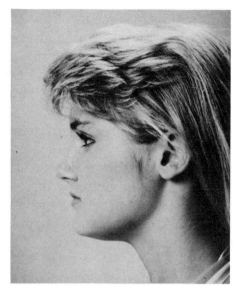

Facial plastic surgery was not the solution for this young girl with a receding chin and thin lips (before, at left). A series of orthognathic procedures over several years improved jaw alignment, and braces expanded dental arches and improved lip definition. The result: the beautiful young lady shown at right.

a small or underdeveloped lower jawbone. In that case, surgery to reposition the jaw may be necessary. This type of surgery, called *orthognathic surgery*, corrects facial bones that have grown incorrectly. An orthognathic surgeon can reposition a poorly aligned jawbone and even lengthen or shorten the upper or lower jaw.

"How is orthognathic surgery done?"

The surgery is usually done in the hospital under general anesthesia, and you may need to stay two or three days. The incisions are made inside the mouth. The surgeon frees the jaw from its attachments and carefully repositions it, moving it either forward or backward as needed, and secures it internally with wires, plates, or screws. The incisions are closed with dissolving stitches.

You will have some swelling and bruising after surgery, but most patients are presentable after a week and can go back to school and resume normal activities. A liquid diet may be necessary at first, but most patients can begin chewing within two weeks after surgery. Healing is usually rapid.

"Will I talk differently afterward if I have jaw surgery?"

Orthognathic surgery doesn't affect the tone and quality of your voice, but it can actually improve speech. This is because people whose jaws and teeth are severely out of line often have speech problems. For instance, people who cannot bring their teeth together are unable to make the "s" sound.

"Does this kind of surgery have any risks?"

Like all surgery, facial plastic surgery is not without risk. Your

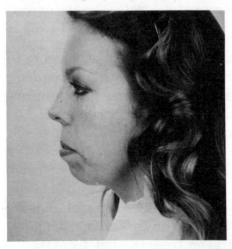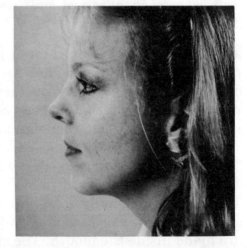

Overcrowded teeth produced the protruding mouth on this young lady (left). Removal of four front teeth and the orthodontic repositioning of the remaining teeth resulted in a more pleasing profile (right). Nasal surgery was performed to bring the nose into harmony with the new chin.

facial plastic surgeon will discuss risks with you at your initial consultation. For instance, there is a small chance of infection. Also, minor asymmetry may occur, requiring a second touch-up procedure.

Small Chin, Big Chin: Augmentation and Reduction Surgery

"I hate my chin," says Sari, 17, "because I don't have one."

Most times the problem is not with the jaw, but the chin bone itself is too small or too large. If you simply have a problem chin, facial plastic surgery may help.

Few people go to a facial plastic surgeon complaining of a weak chin. Usually they go thinking their nose is too big, because the nose may seem to dominate the face of a person with a weak chin. If that is the case, the surgeon can help determine whether the best solution would be a nose job, a chin implant, or both.

"How do they make the chin go out farther?"

A chin implant can be inserted through a small incision made either under the chin or inside the mouth in a procedure called *augmentation mentoplasty*. Local anesthesia and mild sedation are usually used, and healing is quite rapid. The scar is hardly visible. A chin implant can be performed at the same time as a rhinoplasty if both are needed.

"What kind of material is used to get rid of the receding chin, and will it disintegrate someday?"

Chin implants are made of specialized synthetic materials that can be used safely inside the body and do not disintegrate. Implants come in a variety of sizes and shapes, and they can be solid, spongelike, or mesh, depending on the needs of the patient and the preference of the physician.

"I know this girl who has a big chin," points out Todd, 15. *"I wonder if she could do anything to make it smaller."*

"Can anything be done surgically about a turned-up chin?"

The problem of a chin bone that is unusually large is very rare. However, if a big chin bone is the problem, the facial plastic surgeon can make an incision inside the mouth or under the chin and slide the excess bone back.

Nasal Surgery or Chin Implant?

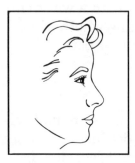 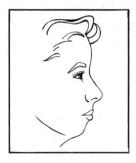 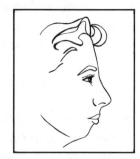

Do you really need nasal surgery? Other facial features can make your nose appear more prominent than it really is. The noses in these three profiles are identical. The face on the left, showing normal jaw structure, presents a pleasing appearance. Notice how the nose appears more prominent when the chin recedes (middle). When a long, sloping forehead is combined with a weak chin (right), the nose seems to project even more.

Excess Fat under the Chin: Liposuction Can Help

"I wish I could do something to get rid of the fat on my chin and throat," comments Katy, 15. "I thought it was baby fat, but it never went away."

If you have ever said this, you may want to know about a technique called *liposuction*. Liposuction, or "fat vacuuming," is a way of removing excess fat cells through a tiny incision in the skin.

Liposuction is definitely not a substitute for losing weight or exercising, but some people have pockets of excess fat cells that no diet or exercise will remove. If a double chin is a family trait, a facial plastic surgeon can help you decide whether liposuction can help.

"Do they remove skin when the face is liposuctioned? If not, wouldn't it sag?"

No. When fat is removed by liposuction in a young patient, the skin contracts and tightens over the area. After the operation, you must wear a snug bandage around your face and neck for a few days or longer, and you may be advised to wear an elastic chin strap at night for several weeks to help the skin contract. Liposuction may be combined with a chin implant in some patients. The operations are done at the same time and through the same small incision beneath the chin.

"Does liposuction hurt? How big is the needle?"

The "needle" is really a *cannula*, a narrow tube no bigger than a soda straw. It is inserted under the skin through a tiny incision beneath the chin. The incision, which is hidden in a natural crease, requires only one or two stitches to close and leaves no visible scar. The surgery, done with local anesthesia and a mild sedative, is

Student Delighted with Chin Surgery

"I feel great about this! It's been fantastic!" says Melanie, of southern Florida. A vivacious college student studying fashion merchandising, Melanie was 19 when she decided to have facial plastic surgery.

"I've always had sort of a baby face," she explains, "but I started thinking seriously about doing something about my face after my jaw was broken in an accident." Her jaw healed eventually, but Melanie had swelling around it for a long time. "It really accentuated the roundness of my face," she recalls.

The swelling eventually went away, but Melanie was left with an acute awareness of her rounded profile. "I realized I had hardly any chin and just too much puffiness under it. After a consultation with a facial plastic surgeon, Melanie decided to have a chin implant and liposuction to remove the fat deposits under her chin. She also asked the surgeon to remove an annoying red mole near her eyebrow.

Melanie had the surgery right in the doctor's office and went home immediately afterward, but she remembers nothing of the surgery. "I couldn't have stood it if I had been aware of what was going on," she says. "It really hurt when I first came out of it, but I took the pain killer my doctor gave me and went to bed for the rest of the day. When I woke up, it was only a little bit sore—not bad at all." Melanie took a week off to recover, but she remembers feeling fine after a few days. "It was good to be able to stay home," she recalls, "because I had to wear this chin strap for a week."

"It was well worth it," Melanie concludes. "I have done a little modeling since having the surgery, and I'd really like to continue with that. Now I have the self-confidence to do it."

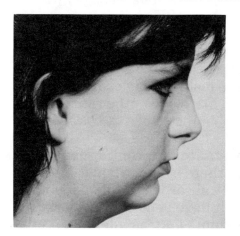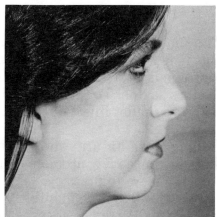

Melanie before, at left, and after chin surgery.

usually without pain, and you will be able to resume your normal activities within three to five days.

"Isn't it dangerous to remove all that fat from under the chin?"

When a facial plastic surgeon uses liposuction, he never removes all the fat from an area. Liposuction is considered extremely safe but, as with all surgery, there is some risk of complications. Among those possible complications are formation of temporary hematomas, or bruising; wrinkling or dimpling of the skin (extremely rare); and temporary paralysis of the nerve in the area that was liposuctioned. Your facial plastic surgeon will discuss these risks with you before you decide to have surgery.

Lips—Is 'Pouty' Better?

"How can I get my lips to look fuller?" asks one teenage girl after another.

The "pouty" look is in—or so say the latest fashion magazines. But is it worth having a surgical procedure to get full, plump, kissable lips—especially when the fashion may change? Many doctors say no. To "plump up" the lips or any other part of the body, you must inject a foreign substance, such as *collagen*.

Collagen is a natural protein substance that comes from calf skin. It causes few problems, but there is one catch: Collagen injections are temporary. The body absorbs the collagen and, within three to nine months, you'll have your old lips back. In a very small number of cases, patients may be allergic to collagen, but this is normally detected before injection through a skin test. Also, temporary lumpiness may result from the injection, but this disappears in time.

The word from here is to leave the plump, pouty look to the fashion models and rely on cosmetics to help you achieve the lips you want. (See chapter 5.)

"How long do the effects of liposuction last? Wouldn't the fat come back as you get older or if you gain weight?"

Fat cells grow bigger as you gain weight, but they don't increase in number once you have matured. Removing pockets of fat like this is considered permanent—once the fat cells are removed they do not come back.

8

... If Your Eyes Droop or Look Angry

"I like my eyes best because they turn different colors depending on what I'm wearing," says Suzanne, 15.

Tim, 17, is even more emphatic: "The eyes are the most expressive part of the face. The best eyes are big and bright, with just the right spacing between them."

What is your favorite facial feature? Which feature best expresses who you are? Many teenagers agree it is the eyes. Your eyes can express your emotions and reflect your deepest feelings. But what if your eyes give a message that is not what you feel?

What if your eyes tilt down at the corners, giving you a droopy look? Or suppose you have heavy, hooded upper lids that make you look stern or angry? Perhaps puffy bags and dark circles under your eyes are making you look tired and dreary. If your problem

goes beyond what can be corrected cosmetically, facial plastic surgery may provide an answer.

Correcting Droopy Eyelids

*"I know some people whose eyes sag a lot. They would look better if
they had eyelid surgery," acknowledges Kim, 16.*

Saggy, drooping eyelids can give you a heavy-lidded look. This can
make it difficult to apply makeup if you are a girl, and can make
people think you look sleepy all the time. In extreme cases, it can
even interfere with your vision.

"Does not getting enough sleep cause droopy eyes?" asks Elaine, 19.

*"My grandmother has these droopy eyes," notes David, 17. "I notice
my little sister has the same eyes. Will she have problems with her
eyes sagging since she has these puppy dog eyes?"*

Not getting enough sleep may make your eyes look tired the next
day, but it won't cause eyelids to droop. Droopy eyes can be hereditary, however, so it is not unusual to see the problem repeated in
family members. If older members of your family have this problem, you may get it also as you age and, when you are older, facial
plastic surgery may help you.

Droopy eyelids are corrected with *ptosis* surgery, which tightens up
the muscle that raises the lid. The incision is made in a natural
crease in the upper eyelid, and because eyelid skin heals so well,
scars are almost never seen.

If your upper eyelids are heavy or appear hooded because of excess
skin, a narrow crescent of eyelid skin can be removed. This operation is called *blepharoplasty*.

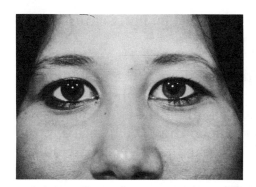 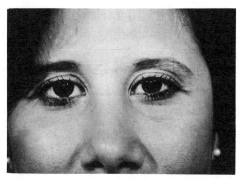

This is an example of a young woman who has a hereditary problem with droopy eyelid folds that cover her eyelids. This condition makes application of eye make-up difficult and ineffective.

"Can they do this surgery to change the eyes of Oriental people?"

Facial plastic surgery can create a double fold eyelid in an Oriental person, but the goal of the surgery is not to make everyone Caucasian. The surgery is useful in eliminating exaggerated features— for instance, some Oriental people have such heavy lids that they can't open their eyes all the way. This can cause fatigue and decreased vision. A facial plastic surgeon will try to reduce the heavy-lidded look without eliminating the person's ethnic identity.

Bags, Circles, and Other Eye Problems
"I get enough sleep, but I always seem to have black circles under my eyes. Is there anything I can do?" asks Sara, 15.

And Maggie, 17, adds, "I'm already starting to get wrinkles under my eyes. My mother has very baggy eyes, too. Help!"

Many people are troubled by dark circles under their eyes. These can have many causes, and often a concealing cosmetic is the only cure. But if the dark circles are accompanied by puffy skin, facial plastic surgery may offer another alternative.

Dark circles under the eyes are often hereditary. The problem is sometimes worsened by puffy skin on the lower eyelids, which can actually cast shadows, making the area under the eyes appear even darker. Bags under the eyes can lend the appearance of premature aging as gravity causes the loose skin to develop wrinkles.

Fat pouches under the eyes can be removed with blepharoplasty on the lower lids. The excess skin is removed through an incision just below the lower eyelid. Scars are barely visible once the incision heals and are usually entirely hidden in natural "smile" lines. However, it is unusual for a teenager to need this type of surgery.

A facial plastic surgeon also can straighten eyes that slant unnaturally by tightening the ligaments that connect the eyelid to the bone. In severe cases, it may be necessary to remove small amounts of bone to bring the eyes into a more natural position.

Having Eyelid Surgery

The skin of your eyelids may be delicate, but it has the ability to heal very quickly with almost no scarring. Eyelid surgery is considered extremely safe when performed by a facial plastic surgeon who does this procedure regularly.

"When you're getting your eyelids fixed, do you see what's happening during the operation?"

No. Eyelid surgery is performed with a local anesthetic along with a medication to help you relax, and you will be only dimly aware of what is going on. The surgery is often done in an office surgery facility, and you will be able to go home shortly afterward. For the "faint of heart," general anesthesia may be used, and an overnight hospital stay may sometimes be required. When the surgery is finished, your doctor may place small sterile strips over the incisions, but your eyes will not be covered. Because your eyelids may swell a little, you may not be able to close them entirely for a few days after surgery.

"Couldn't this kind of surgery damage your eyesight?"

Since facial plastic surgery *is* surgery, it is not without risk. There may be scarring along the eyelid, but this usually is minimal and disappears with time and does not affect vision. In rare instances the eyelid may pull down at the corners. In extremely rare cases, vision may be adversely affected, but the chance of this is almost nonexistent in healthy individuals. It may occur if the patient is diabetic or has high blood pressure, so you should tell your surgeon of any pre-existing conditions that might complicate surgery. After surgery, your vision may seem a little blurry for a day or so, because your surgeon may place an ointment in your eyes to keep them from drying out if your eyelids are swollen. Your surgeon will discuss all of this with you before any surgery is scheduled.

"Does eyelid surgery hurt?"

Some pain should be expected after this type of surgery, but any discomfort is easily controlled with cold compresses and mild pain medication.

"How soon would I be able to go back to school?"

Most people can go back to a normal routine about a week after surgery. You can wear dark glasses for a few days, if necessary, to cover the swelling and to remind you not to touch the area while it is healing. If you wear contact lenses, you should wait two or three weeks before you resume wearing them.

What about Eyelashes and Eyebrows?

"I have a habit of pulling my eyelashes," admits Katy, 14. "I don't pull them out, but I like to tug on them. My mother swears that someday my eyelids are going to swell up. Is that true?"

Yes, this is one of those times that mother knows best. Tugging at the eyelashes can cause tissue damage to the delicate lash hair follicles. This can lead to inflammation that would cause your eyelids to swell. Incidentally, the hair follicles of the eyelashes and the eyebrows are particularly susceptible to damage. Pulling eyelashes out, or excessive brow tweezing, can lead to permanent hair loss.

Connie, 15, wants to shorten her morning makeup routine. "I have heard of some people getting permanent eyeliner put around their eyes," she says. "This sounds like a great way to make putting on makeup easier. Could I have this done?"

Lashliner is actually a type of tattooing, and it is permanent. It is a new technique that is not widely used, but has attracted interest in some circles. However, permanent lashliner has caused problems for some people — such as the pigment moving away from the lashes, loss of the eyelashes, and scarring. While it is considered a relatively safe procedure, some facial plastic surgeons do not recommend this procedure, especially for young people.

9

... If Your Skin Has Scars, Moles, or Birthmarks

"I know a girl who has a birthmark on one entire side of her face," comments Jeremy, 14. *"It makes her look weird to be half and half, so lots of kids won't go near her."*

Sixteen-year-old Chandra's friend has a face problem as well. "His acne was so bad that it left scars on his face, holes really. Can he ever have a smooth complexion again?"

Kate's concern is for her own face. "When I was little," she says, "I had chicken pox, and it left scars on my cheeks and forehead. I always hoped they would go away, but they haven't."

Sixteen-year-old Jan asks, "Is there anything that can be done about moles that are all over the face and look really gross? Some of them even stick out."

And then there's Tiffany, 15, whose skin appears to be several shades of pigment, especially around her eyes and mouth. "Is there anything that can be done besides cosmetics?" she asks.

Although most skin problems clear up with oral medication, topical preparations, and/or cosmetics (see chapters 4 and 5 for details), others do not. Fortunately, facial plastic surgery offers ways to improve many of these facial problems. Teens no longer have to live with pitted, scarred, or stained skin.

Basically there are five ways to treat skin blemishes, scars, and birthmarks: *dermabrasion,* or the sanding of the skin's outer layers; *chemical peel; punch elevation; injectable fillers* that "plump out" pocked areas; and *lasers. Scar revision*, a procedure to make scars from surgery or trauma less visible, is explained in chapter 12.

Dermabrasion Sands the Skin Smooth Again

"I know a guy whose face looks like the surface of the moon, it has so many craters from acne. He'd be so good-looking otherwise," says Shana, 15.

"Do they really use sandpaper to sand the skin away?" asks Robbie, 14. "Doesn't it hurt to have your skin sanded off?"

Dermabrasion can be used to improve acne scars, birthmarks and other areas of excess pigmentation, and raised scar tissue. It is also used to treat severe cases of cystic acne that do not respond to other treatments (see chapter 4). During dermabrasion the surgeon does indeed "sand" off the top layers of the skin, using a rotating brush, however — not a piece of sandpaper. Local anesthetics and topical freezing agents make dermabrasion relatively painless.

Intravenous anesthesia or general anesthesia is used when large areas of the face are treated. The procedure usually is done in the surgeon's office or ambulatory care facility.

If you've ever fallen and skinned a knee, you'll know what your face will look like immediately after dermabrasion. For about 24 hours a yellowish fluid will ooze from the treated area. Some patients experience throbbing or stinging, which is controlled with mild pain relievers and ice compresses. Swelling, ranging from moderate to severe, is usually worse on the second or third day after the treatment and then begins to subside. Depending on dressings used, the treated areas may form crusts, which fall off from one to two weeks after surgery. The new skin will appear very pink for awhile before fading to its normal color over a period of weeks. Excess sun must be avoided to prevent blotchiness and to protect the delicate new skin from burning.

Peeling the Skin Away

For severe acne scarring in young adults, a phenol chemical peel sometimes is used, a procedure whereby a chemical is painted on the skin, which then sloughs away to reveal a clearer layer below. This procedure isn't often recommended for teens, however, because the solution is too harsh for many teens' more delicate skin. Dermabrasion yields better results in young people.

A form of chemical peel known as a "light peel" may be used, however, for some cases of active acne. The skin is painted with trichloroacetic acid and turns white or "frosted" in appearance. The skin later turns red and begins peeling and scaling as the topmost layer falls away. Although complications are rare, some patients do experience a slight variation in skin pigmentation. This usually is related to the patient's originally having very dark pigmentation or going out in the sun too soon after the peel is performed. In some patients, pinkness may persist for awhile, but eventually fades.

Filling in the Grooves

"I'm not sure I would want to go through dermabrasion. Is there any other way to treat my acne scars?" asks Renee, 18.

Comments Eric, 13, "My face would be fine if I didn't have these chicken pox scars."

For acne scarring that is not too deep or widespread, and for the isolated scars that chicken pox often leaves, facial plastic surgeons have two procedures available: punch elevation and injecting special filler materials.

Punch elevation involves the use of a round, circular instrument that is razor sharp. It is used to make a punch incision slightly larger than the scar, cutting a round core. The surrounding tissue is loosened, and the core is pulled up close to the surface of the skin. As the small wound heals, it elevates and presents a smoother appearance in relation to the surrounding skin. If additional smoothness is desired after healing is complete, dermabrasion may be recommended.

Injectable materials include synthetic material, collagen, and certain fats. The filler is injected into the skin with very fine needles. The material fills out the depression, raising it close to the level of the rest of the facial skin. The disadvantage is that injectable fillers are not permanent—the body absorbs the material in time and the procedure must then be repeated. This can occur within six months to a year. However, some people are sensitive to these materials, so a skin test is required before their use.

Chicken Pox Scars No More

"It used to be that I had to put on tons of makeup—I just caked it on," says Justine. "But even that didn't help. In fact, it only made me look worse." Justine describes her problem as "crater face"—the result of a case of chicken pox that she had in the ninth grade.

"I had it really bad, and I couldn't help scratching it," she recalls. "I guess that's the reason I got such deep scars. They were really bad, especially right around my eyes. "I always felt self-conscious. I felt like all everyone could see were these horrible craters."

It never occurred to Justine to have facial plastic surgery. For a long time, she just waited patiently for the scars to get better. Then she tried acne medication, but acne was not the real problem, so that didn't help. Finally Justine's doctor sent her to a dermatologist who recommended surgical treatment. He referred her to a facial plastic surgeon.

"My first thought," Justine recalls, "was 'no way am I going to do that!' " But she decided to go for a consultation. "The doctor was wonderful," she says. "He told us what he could do, showed us pictures, and discussed the cost." Before long, the decision was made. "I had to think a lot about what I was willing to give up," Justine says. "It was the summer before my senior year, and there was a lot going on. I knew I would have to stay out of the sun and miss out on some things. Money wasn't really a problem, since insurance would cover most of it. My family just wanted to do what was best for me. We prayed about it together and decided that, in the long run, it would be worth it. Once the decision was made, I never questioned it at all."

The treatment the facial plastic surgeon used for Justine was a two-step process. The first step, performed in the surgeon's office, was punch elevation—cutting into the deepest scars and actually raising the level of the skin. "That hurt a little," says Justine, who was awake for the procedure. "It felt like he was pulling on my face. I got a little teary-eyed, but he was really concerned about how I was feeling."

After her face healed from the punch elevation, Justine had dermabrasion. "I don't remember anything about it," she says. "The medication he gave me really put me out of it, but I do remember the nurses coming in afterward to check on me and fix my pillows. I had been a little nervous, but I couldn't have asked for a better surgeon."

Afterward, says Justine, "I had a big scab all over my face, and I had to smear it with vegetable shortening four or five times a day until the crusts came off. That was when it started to hurt," she says, adding, "it wasn't terribly painful—more like having a sunburn."

For several months following the dermabrasion, Justine's face was red and she wore a hat outdoors to protect her new skin. "I didn't want to take any chances on messing it up," she says. Her skin now is completely healed, and it looks smooth and natural. "Everybody has some little blemishes," she says. "And that's all I have now! I look natural and I don't wear a lot of makeup. I have my self-confidence back!"

One of the most popular materials for filling in scars and other depressions is collagen, a gel-like substance that is similar to the natural protein of the skin. It is often referred to by the brand names Zyplast® and Zyderm®. Your facial plastic surgeon will decide which kind of injectable filler to use based on your problem and the surgeon's preference.

Laser Therapy—Zap Those Stains Away

"I know a girl who has a big birthmark on her face that makes her lip sort of curl up," notes Marcy, 20. "She acts really aggressive to people, but deep inside I think she's scared to death that no one will like her because of the birthmark."

Jonathan, 19, also knows someone with an unsightly facial mark. "I know a guy who has a birthmark across his face. People think he's been in a bad accident."

Few facial problems cause as much anxiety for young people as do *port wine stains*, those purple birthmarks that result from an overgrowth of enlarged blood vessels in the skin.

Noticeable at birth, port wine stains cause as much anxiety for parents as they do for young people. The typical parental reaction is guilt—mothers often wonder if something done wrong during their pregnancy caused the birthmark.

As the child grows older, other kids frequently stare, ask questions, ridicule, or, perhaps worst of all, turn away in embarrassment. For years there was no recourse but to live with the discoloration, covering it as best one could with makeup such as Dermablend.

What to Do about Moles

An unsightly mole located prominently on the face can be just as devastating as a large acne blemish. Often the mole can be used to advantage. Superstar model Cindy Crawford has perhaps the most famous facial mole in the world next to Elizabeth Taylor's. On both stars, it's considered a beauty mark.

One common treatment for removal of moles that do not appear cancerous is *tangential excision*, a procedure in which the facial plastic surgeon shaves the mole flat with the skin's surface. This leaves a flat scar that is a little whiter than the surrounding skin but more acceptable cosmetically than the mole. A second way to remove moles is by *elliptical excision*, in which the surgeon removes the entire mole, leaving a small and, hopefully, barely noticeable scar.

Excising (cutting out) moles, in rare instances, can have complications. Pitted scars may result and require injectable fillers. Underexcising is more often a problem. In this case, a portion of the mole often remains, and regrowth may occur. If so, the procedure is repeated. More recently, lasers also have been found very effective at removing moles. The procedure used will depend on the type of mole you have and the preference of your facial plastic surgeon.

Young people should be aware that the form of cancer known as *melanoma* is a disease of the young, and, thus, facial moles should be examined for cancerous possibilities. Those that do appear malignant should be excised completely.

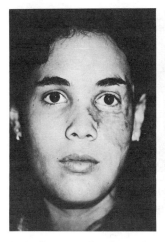 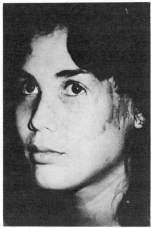 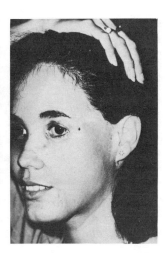

A disfiguring birthmark covered most of this girl's face (left). Through a series of excision operations, her facial plastic surgeon gradually removed the affected skin (center and right).

Laser technology, an effective means to improve port wine stains on adults, has not been used on teens because it produces scarring. But today a new laser provides young people with the same benefit.

Lasers produce intense beams of light and are used for various kinds of surgery. They do not cause pain. The newest version is called a *flashlight-pulsed tunable dye laser*. It uses a yellow light system that passes through ordinary skin harmlessly but is absorbed by anything red. Thus, it is able to "burn away" the enlarged blood vessels of the port wine stain. Since port wine stains affect varying layers of the skin, the number of treatments needed depends on the number of skin layers affected. Skin over bone, for example, requires only half as many treatments as skin over fat. As a rule, the younger the patient, the fewer treatments required.

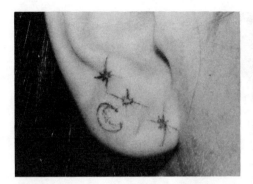 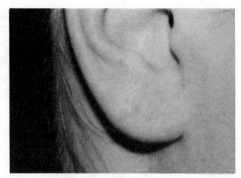

Laser treatment can be beneficial in the removal of tattoos. The young man whose ears are pictured above in "before" and "after" photos had three tattoos removed from his earlobe.

Lasers also can be used to remove other skin abnormalities, such as *spider veins,* or broken capillaries under the skin. Says a skin consultant from California, "Spider veins seem to drive teenagers nuts." These veins, most often found on the nose and cheeks, can be treated effectively with an electric needle that has a needle-nose probe or with a laser. The surgeon places the needle directly into the vein and actually cauterizes the individual vessels, which then close down.

10

. . . If Your Ears Stick Out

"There's a guy in school who has huge ears. He is very self-conscious about them, and a lot of people tease him and call him 'Dumbo,' " notes Jared, 16.

Nancy, 15, confirms that unusual ears are cause for concern. "A girl at work hates to tie her hair back, even though it's required, because her ears stick out."

Flyaway ears. Your parents always thought they were cute. But now you've reached dating age, and names like Mickey Mouse and Dumbo just aren't funny any more. Is there any hope?

If this is your problem, you will be glad to know that the answer is a resounding "Yes!"

Ears may not be anyone's favorite feature, but if yours are mis-shapen, oversized, unbalanced, or protruding, they definitely can be a social liability. Not everyone with prominent ears is bothered by them, but if funny-looking ears are making you miserable, facial plastic surgery can change your outlook.

"I know a guy with funny-looking ears who has a bad temper as a result. Someone called him 'Dumbo' once, and he flew off the handle," reveals Susie, 14.

Teasing can be devastating to a young person's developing personality. For this reason, surgery to correct fly-away or abnormally shaped ears often is done before a child starts school. Since the ears don't do much growing after the age of five or six, ear surgery is one procedure that can be performed safely on young children. But even if you have reached your teen years or your early twenties, it's not too late. The procedure—which surgeons call *otoplasty* —can still be performed successfully. The reason for doing the surgery early is that cartilage is softer then and can be molded more easily.

Why Do I Have These Ears . . . and What Can I Do about Them?

Protruding ears often run in families. Sometimes, the development of the ears stops short in the womb. During early prenatal (before birth) development, the ears stick straight out from the head. As the unborn baby develops, the ears move in closer to the head and develop the natural folds of the normal ear. If the folds do not form, you may end up with cup-shaped ears that stick out from the side of your head. Or you may just have excess cartilage that causes your ears to be too large or sit out too far from your head.

"What exactly do surgeons do to correct ear problems?"

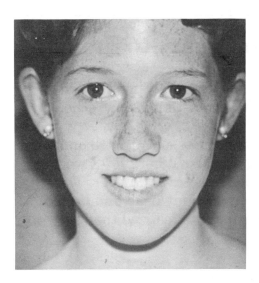 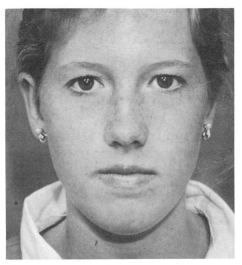

Elana, whose "before" and "after" pictures are shown above, is delighted with the results of her ear surgery. (See story, next page.)

To do an otoplasty, the surgeon makes an incision in back of your ear, removes a small amount of skin, and reshapes the cartilage. If necessary, a few stitches may be placed in the cartilage to create folds that were not there before. Then the incision is sutured to hold the ear until healing takes place and forms scar tissue that will hold the ear in its new position permanently.

"What if one of your ears is bigger than the other? Can they fix one so it looks like the other?"

The major concern in ear surgery is to make the ears as inconspicuous as possible and balanced with the head and facial features. No one has two ears that are identical, and it's not possible to look at both ears at the same time anyway, except from a distance. If one ear sticks out more than the other, the surgery will give you a more balanced look.

Ear Surgery Turns Tears to Smiles

"I used to cry every single morning," recalls Elana. "I don't remember a morning that I didn't cry before I went to school."

Elana isn't crying anymore, and she gets enthused about discussing the surgery that she says changed her life. "I was called 'Dumbo' all through school," she says. "My ears were small, but they stuck straight out from my head and looked terrible." Neither Elana nor her parents realized that ear surgery was possible.

Then the young daughter of a family friend had an otoplasty. "They wanted to save her from years of turmoil like I had been through," Elana says. "I couldn't wait to have it done, too." Elana's family doctor referred her to a facial plastic surgeon.

"The doctor and nurses were great," Elana says. "I was nervous about going in and having everybody stare at my ears and take pictures of them. But the surgeon made me feel comfortable and took plenty of time to answer all my questions. He helped make it a good experience."

"I was terrified before the surgery," Elana says. "I wondered whether it would really work. It was scary to think that my whole image could change, and I might actually be pretty. I was in tears right before they wheeled me in, but the doctor was wonderful about it."

The operation was performed in a local hospital using local anesthesia and intravenous sedation. Says Elana, "I didn't know what was going on, although I did hear music in the background. I felt them nudging my head, but no pain at all."

The first couple of hours after the surgery were "slightly painful, but nothing major," according to Elana. She confesses to a moment of nervousness when the bandages came off the following morning, but says the immediate result looked wonderful.

"I was shocked at the change!" she recalls. "It was so exciting! My ears did look a little puffy and red with some bruising in spots, but healing went really fast. Most of the bruising was gone within a week and a half."

Afterward, Elana says, "I worried about all kinds of strange things—like, would my ears flip back if I went swimming or used a hair dryer?" Actually, one ear did retract slightly, but Elana is not bothered by it. "It's nothing like it used to be, and I'm really not into perfection," she says.

Surgery was definitely worth it, Elana maintains. "No one realizes, unless they have gone through it themselves, how teasing can affect the way you feel about yourself. I felt ugly for years. Even if you have the cutest face in the world, when your ears stick out it's hard to have to wake up every morning and look at them."

"How can they shrink large ears?"

It is not possible to remove cartilage from the tops of the ears safely. But if big ears are too prominent, they can be placed closer to the head, where long hair can hide them more successfully. If your earlobes are excessively long or large, however, facial plastic surgery can make them smaller.

Some Common Ear Concerns

Ear surgery can have dramatic results. It is often performed in the surgeon's office or an ambulatory care facility, and you can go right home afterward.

"Does ear surgery hurt?" "Do you get earaches after this surgery?"

Ear surgery on young adults is usually done with a local anesthetic and intravenous sedation. When performed on young children, general anesthesia may be used. You will be very relaxed and won't feel much sensation while the operation is going on. If you are extremely nervous, your surgeon may prefer to use general anesthesia, which puts you to sleep. This sometimes means spending a night in the hospital. After the surgery, it is typical to have some discomfort for about two or three days, but you won't have an actual earache. Most people who have this surgery have only a small amount of swelling and pain.

"Does ear surgery leave scars?"

Since the incision is made in back of the ear, the narrow scar that results is hidden in the crease behind your ear.

"How soon would I be able to go back to school?"

Special Concerns about Pierced Ears

"I like to wear big earrings. Will my earlobes eventually get stretched out?"

Your earlobes themselves won't get bigger. A more realistic concern is that the holes in your earlobes will enlarge. You may want to give those earlobes a rest periodically. In extreme cases, the earlobe can actually split in two. If this happens, the earlobe can be surgically reconstructed and repierced four to six weeks after surgery.

"I want to have four holes pierced in my ears. Is this okay?"

Multiple holes are not a great idea from a medical standpoint. The biggest danger occurs if the holes are made through cartilage. Infection and actual loss of cartilage are possible. When you get your ears pierced, be sure it is done through the lobe, not the cartilage, and have it done by a doctor who knows how. If you have a tendency to develop keloid (overdeveloped) scars (see chapter 12), ear piercing could present problems.

"Is it possible to get AIDS from trading earrings?"

Not likely. An exchange of blood or other body fluid is needed to transmit the AIDS virus, so there would have to be infected blood on the earring post and an open cut on your ear. A more likely way of getting AIDS is if several people use the same needle to pierce their own ears.

Most people are comfortable going back to school within a week. After surgery, you will wear a soft bandage for a day or two. Your surgeon may ask you to wear a headband or a stocking cap for a week after surgery and keep it on at night for two to four weeks.

"Could ear surgery affect a person's ability to hear?"

No, when it is performed properly, ear surgery has no effect on hearing.

"Are there any complications from this surgery?"

Complications are very rare. All surgery involves risks, however, and you should talk to your surgeon about them. Sometimes, the ear may want to spring back to its former position. This is more likely in people who have the surgery done at an older age, but it occasionally can occur in teens. It can occur to any patient who does not take care to avoid injury to the ear during the first month or so following surgery. If this happens, a second minor tuck-up procedure may need to be done later. In rare instances, infection may occur, requiring the surgeon to remove the stitches and redo the procedure after the infection clears.

11

. . . If Your Cheeks Need Bones

"My face is totally flat," moans Jennifer, 15. "Can facial plastic surgery give me cheekbones?"

Fran, 18, has the opposite problem. "I don't like my cheeks because they are too wide and the cheekbones are too high."

And Christie, 17, speaks for thousands of her peers as she says, "No matter what I weigh, I always have chubby cheeks—the kind that relatives love to squeeze. I just hate that."

There is nothing like great cheekbones to make a face look truly attractive. Just ask any fashion model. But not everyone is born with perfect facial bones. Worse yet, many teens—both boys and girls—are plagued with "chipmunk cheeks." Can facial plastic surgery help?

In this case, the answer is only maybe.

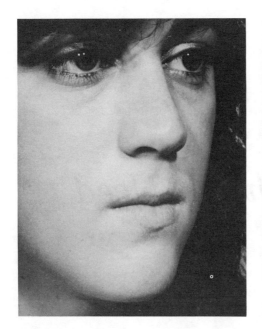 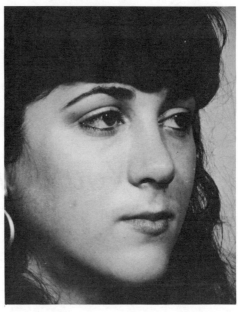

Cheek implant surgery added subtle definition to this young woman's rather thin face as these "before" (left) and "after" photos demonstrate.

Facial plastic surgeons do perform cheek implants to add definition to the face and to help improve facial harmony. The procedure they use is called *malar augmentation*. Cheek implants are sometimes performed along with other facial plastic surgery procedures— such as a rhinoplasty or chin implant—as part of a coordinated program of corrective surgery.

But cheek implants are not for everyone. This surgery is rarely done on teenagers, and almost never before the age of 16. Some surgeons prefer to wait until you reach adulthood, but you may be a candidate for this surgery at age 16 or 17 if you have parental consent, and if you have a serious problem—such as cheekbones that have failed to develop properly.

"How is this surgery done? Where is it done? How long does it take to heal?"

First, the surgeon will study the contours of your face very carefully to determine whether an implant would help you. Some people —for example, those with very little fat under the skin—should not have an implant because it would end up looking like a lump on the cheek. The incision for the implant usually is done either from inside the mouth, between the upper gums and the cheek, or directly under the eye. In each case, the surgeon creates a pocket over the cheekbone and places the implant, closing the incision with a few stitches.

The surgery usually is done with local anesthesia and mild intravenous sedation in the surgeon's office or an ambulatory care facility. Afterward, your face will be somewhat swollen for a few weeks, and it may be difficult for you to chew.

You may experience tightness or numbness around your cheeks that will feel strange while shaving, kissing, or putting on makeup. There normally is not much discoloration with cheek implants, and after a few months you should expect to see an improvement in the way your face looks.

"Are there any complications with cheek implants?"

In some instances, when post-operative swelling has lessened, it may appear that the implants are asymmetrically placed. If this occurs, the implants will be repositioned after a number of months. The patient must avoid injury to the cheeks, as the implants can move during the first month or so after surgery.

Computer-assisted Imaging Lets You See Facial Changes

Imagine if you could look into a crystal ball and see what you may look like in a few years. What if you were given an advance picture of what facial plastic surgery could do for you? Many surgeons are now using a new technology that makes this possible.

Using a computer, high-resolution monitor, video camera, special software, and an electronic sketch pad, the facial plastic surgeon can display your image on the screen and then change any of your features using a lightpen or "mouse." The surgeon can even "age" your face to show you the difference two or three years might make.

Sometimes, just seeing how you may change in another year or two can help you accept a temporary problem like "chipmunk cheeks." Maybe you won't need surgery! If you do, computer-assisted imaging can help you and your surgeon decide what should be done—without actually doing it.

Even if you are not yet old enough for surgery, it may be tremendously reassuring for you to know that help is possible and to get an idea of what you may look like eventually. Seeing how your face may change and knowing what can be done through facial plastic surgery may make it easier for you to wait until the appropriate age for surgery.

How accurate is computer-assisted imaging? The computer cannot take into account such things as your underlying bone and muscle structure and your capacity to heal. But it can simulate maturation and surgical changes with a high degree of accuracy.

Not all facial plastic surgeons use computer-assisted imaging, and not all of those who do have the software to "age" your face. Some feel that computer imaging gives patients a false guarantee of surgical results. So be sure you understand that while it is highly accurate, computer-assisted imaging is not a guarantee of your actual results.

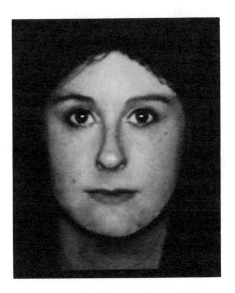 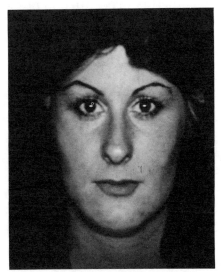

The computer screen above left shows a patient as she appears today. The screen at right suggests her appearance ten years from now. Teens may be gratified to learn that their chubby cheeks will thin down with age.

"What if your cheekbones are too high?"

This problem is fairly rare, but if excessively high cheekbones are interfering with facial harmony, they can be modified. The procedure is very similar to implant surgery, except that the surgeon will remove a small amount of the excess bone through the incision rather than insert an implant.

"What about very chubby cheeks? Can facial plastic surgery make your face thinner?"

Some surgeons perform cheek liposuction (a procedure for vacuuming out excess fat deposits through a small incision), but most agree that this procedure is not appropriate for teenagers.

It may help to know that your face is going to continue to change into your early twenties. As your facial features mature, your face will narrow and you may well lose those excess fat deposits. If you have the fat removed at too early an age, you may end up with a really ugly indentation in your face after you mature.

"But I really hate my round face! Isn't there any hope for me?"

A facial plastic surgeon can analyze the features of your face to determine whether it is possible to change their proportions. For instance, if your face is too round, it may be that you have a very short jaw. If so, a chin implant may make your face look longer. You may be helped by surgery to add cheekbones, and certain changes to your nasal structure also can help to elongate your face. Also, see chapter 5 for cosmetic tips on making your cheekbones appear more prominent.

IV

Disfiguring Accidents and Diseases

12

Accidents, Injuries, and Lingering Scars

*"A friend of mine was playing football and ran into a mailbox,"
says Karen, 15. "He had to have 88 stitches on his face. When I first
saw him after it happened, he had a lot of scars, but he's had facial
plastic surgery several times, and now he looks a lot better than he
did at first. He still has to have more surgery."*

*"A kid I knew fell off the side of a retaining wall and really messed
up his face. His chin and jaw still look crooked," notes Peter, 14.*

*Amy, 19, points out an all-too-common injury scenario for young
people. "Several of my friends have been in car accidents and have
scars on their faces. They say they can't have surgery for at least a
year. Why is that?"*

*"There's a mean dog in our neighborhood, and I'm always scared
he'll jump on me and bite my face," says Beth, 12. "It happened to
one kid already."*

Skateboard Mishap Crushes Face

Craig doesn't remember anything about the accident that left his face crushed. "I was lying down on a skateboard going down a hill," he says. "It was dark, and there was a parked car. I don't really know any more about it."

The details are filled in by Craig's mother and his surgeon. The skateboard probably achieved a speed of 50 miles per hour as Craig flew down the hill, they estimate. He hit the car with his upper jaw, crushing his nose and rolling his face back.

"Nothing was left of the inside of his nose," says his mother. "The surgeon found tissue from his nose pushed up between his eyes and performed surgery to bring it back down. He had to remove paint chips from the car that were embedded in Craig's face. He had to rebuild his nose, graft bone to replace his upper jaw, and implant four new upper teeth."

Corrective surgery, some of it intensely painful, took years. Because of injuries to Craig's brain, general anesthesia was out of the question, and Novocain® was inadequate. "It was horrible for him, but he had unbelievable courage," his mother maintains. "His attitude was excellent, and that really is what pulled him through."

Craig was able to return to high school after the major injuries healed, but it was years before his appearance started to return to normal. "I didn't have my upper teeth for a couple of years," he recalls. "Sometimes that got to me. I couldn't smile

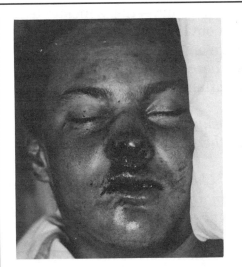 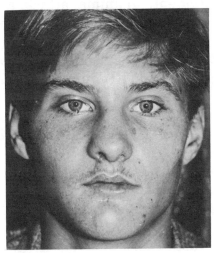

Even though a skateboard accident crushed Craig's face, "before" photo at left, facial plastic surgery made him look normal again, right.

or talk to girls without it showing. But I really didn't think about it too much. My friends stuck by me. Other people would stare, but I just didn't let it bug me."

Today, Craig says, "I don't even have scars. The doctor did a great job. It was really a miracle." Does he look the way he used to? "I don't remember," he says.

Craig's rebuilt nose will always be somewhat crooked. Sometimes people ask him if it has ever been broken. "We notice the difference," says his mother, "but people don't look twice at him. His appearance is normal."

Meanwhile, Craig is busy getting on with his active lifestyle. He doesn't worry about his appearance. "I'm easy," he says.

An accident, an animal attack, a sports injury—these incidents are always traumatic. Being left with an obvious scar on the face, missing tissue, or damaged bone structure only adds to the emotional distress. But you should know that there is much a facial plastic surgeon can do to minimize or camouflage facial injuries.

"I would be very interested in plastic surgery if I were in an accident. I don't think I'd be interested otherwise," says Andy, 17.

Robyn, 16, has a similar attitude: "If I had a serious disfigurement caused by a birth defect, or if I were in an auto accident and got my face messed up—I think I'd want to have facial plastic surgery."

The vast majority of teens are fairly satisfied with the way they look. But almost all are concerned about what could happen if an accident occurs. Facial plastic surgery is much more than just cosmetic improvement—many people need this type of surgery to restore normal appearance and function after an injury. Facial plastic surgery techniques also are used to correct severe birth defects.

The field of facial plastic surgery developed rapidly during World War I when doctors began to see a need to help young soldiers whose faces had been shattered during trench warfare along the Western Front in France. The techniques used then have since been refined and improved.

While no one can guarantee that the victim of a serious accident will look exactly the same as before, facial plastic surgery can do much to restore a more normal—even attractive—appearance to people who have experienced severe facial injury.

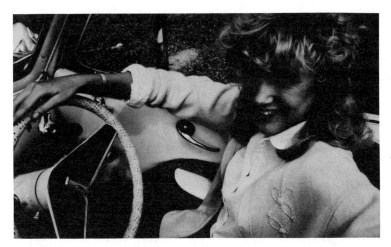

Although young people look forward with great anticipation to the day they get their driver's license, automobile accidents cause facial injuries in far too many young people each year.

First Stop: The Emergency Room

"If my face is cut in an accident, will there be a facial plastic surgeon in the emergency room?"

The care you get immediately after an accident can affect the way you will look after you heal. If you have a facial injury, you probably will be cared for by surgeons who specialize in reconstructive surgery of the face. In many small community hospitals it is common practice to transport victims of serious accidents to large regional medical centers, where their wounds can be treated by experienced specialists.

Any time there is a serious injury involving the bones of the face, particularly the jaw, the nose, or the bones surrounding the eyes, it is wise to have a facial plastic surgeon on the treatment team. Minor injuries needing only stitches often are handled by emergency room physicians or a family doctor, but when the injury crosses the lip, eyelid, eyebrow, or nostril, you or your parents may want to request a facial plastic surgeon who specializes in facial reconstruction.

Softball Plays Havoc
with Young Player's Nose

Brittany would rather forget the accident that sent her to the hospital for reconstructive surgery, but she is glad that a facial plastic surgeon was on hand five years ago to repair the damage.

Brittany was 10 years old at the time. It was the first day of softball practice, and it was raining. Brittany was warming up by pitching to her coach when he lobbed in a pop fly. "I lost the ball," Brittany relates. "It was a white softball and it just blended in with the clouds and the sky and the rain. The next thing I knew, there was blood all over my face. I didn't even feel it hit. I guess I was in shock."

Brittany's nose was shattered, but no one realized that right away. In fact, her coach didn't even believe it was broken. In the emergency room, a staff physician stitched up the cut on Brittany's nose. Then, another doctor looked at it and expressed concern that the stitches would leave a visible scar. He suggested calling in a facial plastic surgeon, who immediately removed the original stitches and did the job over in a way that would minimize scarring.

Because her nose was so swollen, it was not apparent right away how badly damaged the bone was. Brittany was released from the hospital, but she experienced trouble breathing and constant pain. A couple of weeks later, she was back in the hospital. This time the facial plastic surgeon performed surgery to reconstruct her shattered nasal bones.

Although Brittany was asleep for the surgery, she remembers waking up in pain. Her nose, she recalls, "looked awful—it was even more swollen than it was right after the accident, and I had black eyes and bandages all over my face." After three days in hospital, Brittany went home to complete her recovery. "When I went back to school, the other kids stared at me a lot, but everyone was sympathetic," she says.

About two weeks later, Brittany had the stitches inside her nose removed. She remembers that the swelling took several weeks to go down and she had black eyes for at least a month. But that was just a minor inconvenience. The good news is that Brittany's nose healed perfectly. And how does it look now? "Exactly the same as it did before the softball hit me," she says in a pleased voice.

"Exactly what will the doctors do to save my face if I've gone through the windshield of a car?"

There are two stages to repairing serious facial injuries. First, injuries to the bones of the face are dealt with; then the doctor turns his attention to covering areas where skin or tissue has been lost or damaged. Afterward, it is often necessary to do follow-up procedures to improve the appearance of the face and reduce scarring. For more on scars, see chapter 9.

When the Injury Is More than Skin Deep

"I've heard about people who have their jaws or face wired together after an accident. What does this mean?"

"If the bones truly are shattered in an accident, is there any way the person will look normal again?"

If bones are broken, the surgeon realigns the fragments, being careful to restore proper function. Function always comes first. The surgeon starts by reconstructing the "bite" of the jaws and then concentrates on repairing the rest of the facial skeleton. Fractures around the eye receive special attention so that the eye itself maintains its proper position. Final appearance is an important consideration, but it is even more important for the jaws, nose, and eyes to function properly.

Facial fractures are often repaired with *miniplates*—a new technique in which small, thin strips of metal are used to hold the bones together. Tiny screws secure the plates permanently in place. A broken jaw, for example, may be wired to hold it in position, but if actual loss of bone has occurred, the surgeon may graft on bone and secure it with a miniplate. Bone often is borrowed from the outer layer of the skull or from the hip bone. The layer of bone removed from the skull regenerates, so the skull eventually regains its normal thickness.

"A friend of mine was in an accident several years ago and now she looks very strange on one side of her face. They had to build up her jaw and cheek. It looks sort of flat and very unattractive. She's pretty on the other side," comments Melanie, 14.

Most bone problems are taken care of immediately after an accident, but broken bones don't always heal evenly. When facial bones are badly shattered, the surgeon may need to allow Mother Nature time to let the wound heal before attempting to reposition them. When bones don't heal properly, surgeons may use a plastic implant to restore facial symmetry. For example, if an injury has

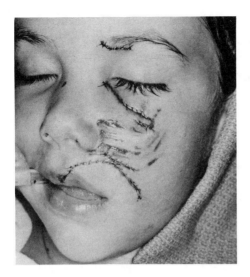 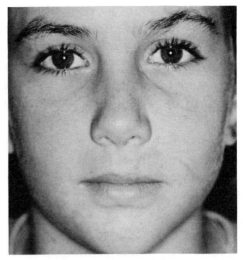

When a Doberman bit Dora, her lip was so badly torn you could see her teeth. In the emergency room, a facial plastic surgeon performed an immediate repair of her facial lacerations (left). Four years later (right), after scar revision surgery, Dora's injury is barely noticeable.

made one cheek a little flatter than the other, a cheek implant may help. This operation is done essentially the same way as a cosmetic cheek implant (see chapter 11). But surgeons can actually carve the implant to customize it for the patient's needs, or even use a computer to design a customized implant. Plastic implants can replace shattered bones in the jaw and head areas as well.

"My friend tried to break up a cat fight when he was younger, and he was clawed so badly that part of his ear came off," notes Brad, 13. *"He looked ruined. He got stitches, but he still looks strange."*

Surgeons are sometimes called upon to try to reconstruct damaged ears and noses. These are among the most challenging problems a facial plastic surgeon faces.

While it may not be possible to restore the patient's original appearance, advanced grafting techniques have made it possible for surgeons to rebuild these features using cartilage and skin taken from other parts of the body. For instance, when bone or cartilage is lost from the nose, it can be repaired by grafting a small amount of cartilage taken from the ear. The nose is rebuilt, and then the ear is repaired and restored to a normal appearance. When the injury is extensive or severe, more than one operation may be required. It may take months or even years to complete the entire process.

Repairing Skin Injuries

"What if so much of the skin is lost that it can't be pulled back together again?"

Minor skin injuries usually heal with little problem, but when large areas of skin are lost, the skin cannot regenerate. One way to repair the damage involves *skin flaps,* or lifting a flap of skin from a nearby area and swinging it into position to cover the injury. Because the donor skin is never entirely separated from its blood supply, skin flaps work better than grafts for treating these types of injuries.

A flap of skin is cut out in a geometric pattern, leaving one side of the flap attached. Surgeons use a variety of designs, depending on the part of the face involved and the extent of the injury. The flap is then rotated and stitched into its new position, and the edges of the donor site are brought together and closed.

What if the skin in the donor area is too tight to close up? Or suppose there is not enough undamaged skin left to cover the injured area? One possible answer is *tissue expansion*. Surgeons can use tiny balloon-like devices to stretch areas of healthy skin. The balloons are implanted under healthy tissue and are slowly expanded by injecting sterile water at regular intervals into the balloons. In this way the healthy skin is gradually stretched. After about six weeks, the balloons are removed and a skin flap is made from the expanded skin. This expansion also may be done at the time of surgery, without the six-week wait, depending on the amount of expansion needed and the surgeon's preference. When tissue expansion is used for treatment of large scars, the scarred area is excised (cut out), and the newly stretched skin is repositioned to cover the damaged area. The facial plastic surgeon will try to make the remaining narrow scars fall into natural creases of the face, if possible, so that they will not be as noticeable. (For more uses of tissue expanders, see chapter 14.)

Repairs of this type usually require extended hospitalization, especially when large areas of skin are lost. The treatment may require numerous procedures, performed in stages over a long period of time. Once the major wounds have healed and the patient is released from the hospital, some of the remaining surgeries may be done on an outpatient basis. A hospital stay may be required if general anesthesia is used.

Scars Often Can Be Minimized

"Two girls in our school were in a car accident, and they may need facial plastic surgery," relates Brian, 17. "One has a scar that goes from ear to ear across her face. It's hard not to stare at it. I feel sorry for her. Can anything be done about it?"

Scar tissue forms any time the skin is cut all the way through. It is important to understand that once you have a scar, it will be there forever. Scars cannot be erased or removed. The goal of scar revision surgery is not to remove scars, but to change their shape or position in order to camouflage them more successfully.

Prevention Is the Best Cure

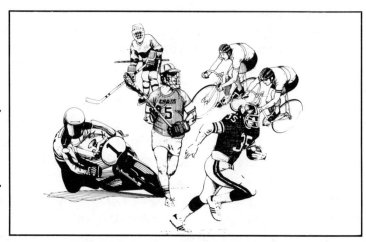

You don't have to have an automobile accident or other major trauma to end up with scars. Even minor injuries can leave visible scars if they are not treated properly. Although facial plastic surgery can do much to improve unsightly scars, there are two even better techniques: (1) prevent serious injuries in the first place, and (2) minimize scarring by proper wound care.

Preventing Serious Injuries

Always wear a seatbelt whenever you are in an automobile, even if it is just a short trip. Many severe facial injuries are the result of striking the dashboard, steering wheel, or windshield. Even a minor accident at low speed can cause a facial injury if you are not wearing a seatbelt.

Always use proper protective equipment when you play contact sports. Be sure to wear a well-fitting helmet, face guard, or mouth protection whenever appropriate.

Invest in protective safety glasses if you engage in potentially dangerous activities (especially if you wear hard or gas-permeable contact lenses). Wear appropriate protective eye-wear to play racquetball, when using power tools, or while working in a chemistry laboratory.

Be especially careful when playing sports that do not require protective equipment. Facial plastic surgeons report that more facial injuries occur from basketball, softball, and base-ball than from football.

Proper Wound Care

If an injury occurs, get appropriate first aid immediately. Wounds have to be cleaned thoroughly, particularly if there is a chance that dirt particles have gotten into them. Dirt or grit embedded in a wound can permanently tattoo the skin.

Get stitches if the cut seems deep. If the cut is on your face, you may want to have a facial plastic surgeon do the stitching. The doctor's expertise can make a big difference in how well the wound heals. If the skin is scraped, keep it clean and covered.

Research has found that "moist healing" can actually cut heal-ing time in half by preventing a scab from forming. This meth-od can also reduce scarring. Flexible, waterproof bandages that can even stay on during bathing are available at drug stores.

Even a narrow scar can attract unwanted attention, especially if it goes in a straight line that crosses the natural lines of the face. Scars that form a J or U shape also can be particularly troublesome. Fortunately, these types of scars often respond well to scar revision surgery.

One way to correct straight line scars is through a technique called a *geometric broken line closure*. The surgeon camouflages the line of the scar by breaking it up into a tiny geometric pattern of little triangles and squares. Because the new scar is irregular, it doesn't catch the eye the way a straight line does. It blends in with the natural skin texture and is much less noticeable.

A similar technique, called the *running W-plasty*, involves breaking up a straight scar by cutting a row of tiny W or Z shapes into the scar tissue. When this heals, the new scar often disappears into the natural lines and creases of the face. Surgeons generally use the running W-plasty on vertical scars.

"I have two scars on my face from a three-wheeler accident, and they drive me crazy," notes Elizabeth, 19. "They're so wide that nothing will hide them. Can facial plastic surgery help me?"

Possibly. Wide scars are sometimes improved by excision, which means simply cutting the scar tissue out and bringing the edges together. The goal here is to replace a wide scar with a narrow one. Another method used for very wide scars is to improve the scar a little at a time over a period of months. After each procedure, the remaining skin is stretched and the incision closed. After this heals, a little more of the scar is improved, until all that remains is a narrow line. Scars can be minimized through several other procedures, including dermabrasion and injectable fillers. See chapter 9 for details.

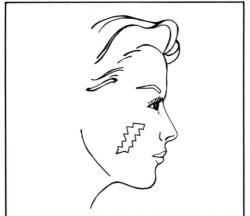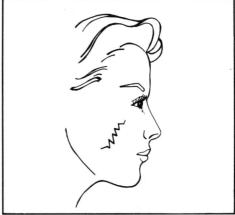

Excising a section of acne scarring on the cheek using a double row of tiny **W** *shapes helps to make the resultant scar appear less obvious.*

Other Types of Scars

"I know someone who had a bad cut near his lip," points out David, 14. "The scar is bad enough, but it also seems to pull his lip up on one side. Can they do anything to make him look normal?"

Sometimes when an injury runs into an open area such as a lip, eyelid, or nostril, the scar can tighten as it heals, pulling the facial features out of place. This problem is called a *contracted scar.*

Contracted scars can be released with a procedure called *Z-plasty.* The goal of this procedure is to make the scar a bit longer, so that it does not pull the skin. The surgeon cuts along the original scar and then makes two additional cuts above and below it at angles to form a **Z.** The two small flaps of skin are readjusted and carefully stitched, resulting in a smooth, narrow scar that does not pull the skin.

Annette, 16, poses this question: "I know someone who has a really large scar that seems to be getting bigger. Why would it do that?"

Overdeveloped scars that continue to enlarge are called *keloid scars.* The tendency to develop keloid scars seems to run in families, and they are found more in black and other dark-skinned people than in whites. Keloids are most likely to develop in the earlobes, chin, and neck. (Those with a tendency to develop keloid scars should be wary of ear piercing — see chapter 10.)

Keloid scars are often improved by excision. Injections of cortisone and laser treatment may also be used. Usually only a small scar remains after surgery for keloid scars. Be sure to let your facial plastic surgeon know if anyone in your family has developed keloid scars in the past.

Who Should Have Scar Revision Surgery?

If you have been troubled for years by an unsightly scar, consultation with a facial plastic surgeon who is experienced in scar revision can help you determine whether this type of surgery can help. On the other hand, if you have recently suffered an accident, time may be the best healer, but you should consult a facial plastic surgeon early so that your particular healing processes can be monitored.

"I have a friend who ran his moped into a barbed wire fence. He was cut across the middle of his face and it's all swollen and black and blue. Will he need facial plastic surgery?" asks Kyle, 15.

No one can predict the final appearance of a scar. In fact, scars usually get worse before they get better. It can take anywhere from six months to two years for a scar to reach its final state.

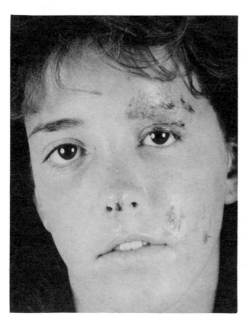 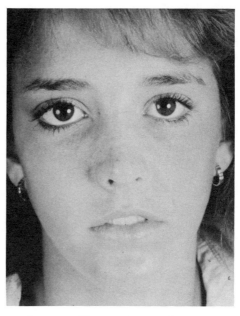

Surgery is not the only way to improve scars. Given sufficient time and proper care, scars may disappear by themselves, as occurred with this young woman. Mother Nature's ability to heal is one reason facial plastic surgeons often recommend waiting for six months to a year before seeking surgery to improve scars.

Whenever the skin is cut, tiny new blood vessels are formed in the area to help speed healing. This causes the whole area to look red. As the edges begin to heal, collagen fibers are laid down, making the new scar look raised and lumpy. This stage may last up to six weeks. Finally, the scar begins to soften and shrink. This process may continue for a year or more. Often the passage of time can reduce an unsightly scar to the point that it is barely noticeable. That is why doctors recommend waiting until the scar has completely matured before seeking scar revision surgery. So even though you may want a facial scar fixed immediately, don't be impatient!

13

Burns

"A coffee pot fell on my brother when he was little, and he still has an ugly scar across the side of his face where he was burned," relates Kurt, 19. "Will he ever be able to get rid of it?"

"My girlfriend got burned when her hair caught on fire after she put gasoline on a camp stove fire," says Barb, 16. "She's been in the hospital for surgery several times, but her face and scalp are still a mess."

Few scars are as unattractive and difficult to camouflage as a burn scar. Severe burns can destroy several layers of skin and leave the healed area reddened or bumpy. While burn scars are difficult to treat, there are facial plastic surgery techniques that may help to reduce the scarred area.

Today, people who have serious burn injuries often are treated in comprehensive burn centers where specialists handle all aspects of the healing process, from the immediate treatment through the final skin grafts. These centers use modern techniques that can minimize scarring. Even people who suffered a burn injury several years ago may be able to be successfully treated today.

"I know a guy who caught on fire, and at the hospital they put pig skin on the burnt places," relates Michael, 18. "The guy looks terrible. Could a doctor fix his complexion?"

It is very important to get the burned area covered quickly—when large areas of the body are left without skin, infection and severe pain are unavoidable. Depending on the extent of the burns, the patient may not have adequate amounts of healthy skin for the doctors to graft onto the burned area. Pig skin and other human skin are sometimes used to cover burned areas temporarily. In addition, a new synthetic skin has been developed that helps improve coverage during the natural healing process.

Scar revision surgery can often help an individual left with unattractive burn scars. How much can be done depends on the depth of the burns, how extensive they were, whether enough healthy skin is available, and how much the scars have contracted.

"Are scars from burns any different from scars sustained in an automobile crash?"

Most of the techniques used to reduce accident scars are also used for burn scars. Small areas of scarring sometimes can be excised, or cut out. When the scarred area is extensive, grafting of healthy skin from another part of the body may help to improve the appearance of the scar. Dermabrasion, or facial sanding, is not a possibility with burn scars because skin that has been burned is too delicate to sand.

"Where does the skin come from for grafting to cover scars?"

Surgeons try to take skin from areas where it is not really needed or where it will not show. For example, some people have a lot of loose skin around their upper eyelids. If this is the case, some of this skin may be removed and used as a skin graft. Skin may also be taken from behind the ear or from some other location.

Tissue expansion also is used for treating burn scars. If there is not enough healthy skin to use for grafting, surgeons can slowly stretch the skin with small balloons implanted under the skin adjoining the burned area. Then the surgeon cuts out the scarred area and stitches the edges of skin together. This technique is particularly helpful for burn scars on the face, because all that is left is a narrow scar that often can be hidden in a natural crease. (For more on tissue expansion, see chapters 12 and 14.)

"Will there be scarring in the area the skin graft is taken from?"

Yes, scars will remain both in the area that skin is removed from and in the area of the graft. The surgeon will try to camouflage the remaining scars in natural folds of skin or take the graft from an area that normally is covered by clothing.

"What if the skin taken from another part of your body for grafting is a different color than your face?"

Grafted skin often is a different color or texture. The surgeon will try to select skin from an area that closely matches the color and texture of the burned area, but this is not always possible when a person is burned over a large area.

New Hope for Burned Scalps

It was a roundabout path that led Danny to have scalp flap surgery. "When I was about 18 months old, I was burned pretty severely when hot oil from frying chicken spilled on my head. The burns healed, but I was left bald all down the right side of my head."

Danny tried three different transplant operations at various times, but all were unsuccessful. Finally he gave up and re-signed himself to having long hair from the other side of his head parted to grow down over the bald area. "It didn't really show — unless the wind blew," he says. "Still, I always wor-ried about the way I looked. I just wasn't happy with it."

Danny was a junior when his mother met a facial plastic sur-geon who told her about a new procedure being performed on the West Coast. She encouraged Danny to talk to the doctor, and what he heard made him eager to try again. So during the summer after his junior year in high school, Danny trav-eled to California where he learned he was an ideal candidate for *scalp flap surgery*. (See chapter 14 for more on hair re-placement surgery.) The facial plastic surgeon implanted a tissue expander under his scalp. Then Danny returned home to Colorado, where he visited a local surgeon three times a week to have sterile water injected into the expander.

"I had to wear a hat all that summer," laughs Danny. "It just kept growing, and it was uncomfortable at times." Danny re-members getting a bad headache after each injection, but it didn't last long. The device stayed in place for six weeks, then Danny went back to California to have the surgery.

"The operation was one of the more interesting experiences of my life," Danny says. "I wasn't really asleep the whole time— I could hear people talking, and I knew they were putting the staples in my scalp." Danny says he felt no pain at all during the operation, "just fear—a lot of fear!" He continues: "They had an instant camera right there in the waiting room, and the first thing they did after they were done was take a picture and hand it to me. It was pretty amazing. I was happy about it right away. Suddenly I had hair growing normally all over my head!" Nothing really changed for Danny after the surgery. "It's not like people had been teasing me or making comments. It was more my own insecurity. The best part of having surgery is that now I just don't think it about it anymore."

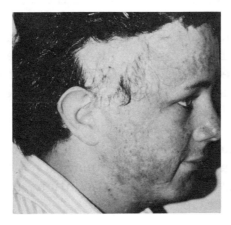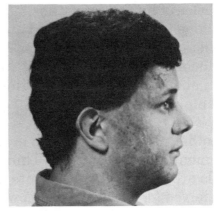

Danny before scalp flap surgery (left) and after (right), with his hair growing normally.

"What if the skin used for grafting is from an area where hair grows? Will hair grow on your face?"

If only the very top layers of skin are used for the graft, then no hair will grow because the hair follicles are not taken. If the burn is deep, and it is necessary to take the full depth of skin from a hair-bearing area like a leg or the chest, then hair will grow on the grafted area. Surgeons do not do anything to destroy the hair follicle because it is so important to protect the blood supply of the skin taken for grafting. After healing is complete, the person can have *electrolysis* to eliminate the unwanted hair permanently (see chapter 14).

"I know a boy who is rather cute, but he is a fireman and his face was burned," comments Jennifer, 20. "He doesn't have any noticeable scars, but when he lets his whiskers grow, there is a small patch where nothing grows. Why?"

The burn was deep enough to do permanent damage to the hair follicles of his face and, thus, hair no longer will grow. Nothing can be done to restore damaged hair follicles. In the beard, however, revising the scar by narrowing it might improve the appearance by reducing the non-hair-bearing area on the face. For more information about treating burn injuries in places where hair grows, see chapter 14.

Another use of skin grafts is in the treatment of vitiligo, the lack of pigmentation on the skin. Thin layers of skin with normal melanin cells are grafted onto the white areas. Nonsurgical solutions are preferred for young people, however (see chapter 5).

14

Too Little or
Too Much Hair

"There is a guy who sits in front of me in class who has something wrong with the hair on the back of his head," comments Natalie, 13. "He has a big bald spot, and the skin there is lumpy and strange looking."

"I have long hair that has always been thick and full," says a very worried-sounding Janine, 16. "Lately, though, it seems to be falling out almost in clumps. What's wrong with me?"

"Hair is the one thing that gives guys a real sense of individuality," declares Marc, 19. "No wonder we worry about it so much."

Hair is second only to complexion as an object of concern when teens consider the state of their appearance. Most worry more about the manageability of their hair than its actual loss, but for those few who do have hair loss problems, the impact on their self-esteem can be critical. The good news for those who are missing

hair is there are some solutions at hand. Basically there are three
causes of hair loss: injury, hormonal problems, and disease, specifically the immunological disorder known as *alopecia areata*. Extreme dieting, stress, pregnancy, chemotherapy (radiation treatment for certain cancers), and illness also can cause hair loss, but
usually the hair grows in again three to four months after the
cause has ended. For a small group of teens, the problem is too
much hair—not too little—usually the result of a hormonal
imbalance.

New Hope for Major Scalp Injuries

Childhood burns—the kind that occur when a toddler pulls a pot
off the stove—are one of the biggest causes of hair problems in
teenagers. Accidents that tear away part of the scalp and surgical
removal of tumors on the head also can cause permanent hair loss.
Although this type of problem is not widespread, it can be devastating if it happens to you.

As recently as a few years ago, there was no practical way to replace hair lost because of injuries or surgery. Today, some revolu-
tionary new techniques make hair replacement possible for some
young people.

*"What can a facial plastic surgeon do if you have lost a lot of hair in
an automobile accident or from some other kind of head injury?"*

As long as there are some undamaged areas remaining on the
scalp, a facial plastic surgeon may be able to use the existing hair
to cover the damaged areas.

The first step is a technique called tissue expansion. The surgeon
will stretch the healthy, hair-bearing scalp by implanting a small,
deflated balloon under the skin. Twice a week for several weeks,

the person returns to the doctor's office to have sterile water injected into the balloon. As the balloon expands over a period of time, the skin stretches. Because it happens so gradually, there is very little discomfort—but the patient does have to put up with the growing bulge on his or her scalp.

When the healthy scalp has been stretched enough, the surgical part of the treatment—scalp flap surgery—begins. Incisions are made, and a portion of the healthy scalp is partially separated. An area of bald scalp is removed, and the newly stretched flap of hair-bearing scalp is rotated into position to cover the damaged area. The flap is stitched into place and the edges of healthy scalp are pulled together and stitched shut. The whole process may require several surgical procedures. In many cases, surgeons may be able to reconstruct the hair so that it looks almost normal.

What about Premature Baldness?

It is very rare to see visible signs of balding in teenage boys. But some teenage boys have noticed a thinning hairline.

Nearly two-thirds of all men eventually become bald, and about 25 percent will have noticeable thinning by the time they reach their mid-twenties. If early baldness runs in your family, it is possible that you are noticing the earliest sign of what doctors call *male-pattern baldness*. What happens is that the hair follicles on the head are pre-programmed to be sensitive to androgens (male hormones) and will fall out when androgen levels rise sufficiently high. Although much rarer, because these hormones also are present in females in small quantities, this problem can manifest itself in girls, too.

However, don't panic unnecessarily. Baldness in men is hereditary, but the trait can be passed on by either your mother or your father,

Accident Rips Away Girl's Scalp

It was her 15th birthday, and Loni and her three friends were thinking only of the school dance they had just left. It was foggy, and the driver of the little MG convertible was following the lines on the side of road. "We came to the access to the highway, and he didn't see it and ran up over a guardrail," Loni explains. "The car flipped over and slid about 500 feet, and I guess my head went through the convertible top."

Loni and her friends had to be cut out of the car and were rushed to the emergency room, where a facial plastic surgeon immediately took over Loni's care. She recalls being conscious the whole time, saying, "The accident must have affected the nerves in my head, or maybe I was in shock, because I could not feel a thing. I was covered with blood, but I didn't feel scared, just worried about my parents' reaction. I do recall wondering if I would ever have a normal head again."

Loni had reason to worry. A section of scalp about four inches long had been ripped away. Several surgeries were needed to close the wound and restore her appearance. First, the surgeon rotated flaps from other parts of her scalp to cover the damaged area. Then skin was taken from behind her ear and grafted to cover the open area that remained.

That still left her with a large scarred area on the side of her head and a noticeable bald spot. The facial plastic surgeon improved as much of the scar as possible a little bit at a time —a procedure called *serial excision*. Then, when Loni's scalp couldn't be stretched anymore, he filled in the remaining bald area with *punch grafts*—hair transplants taken from the thick hair on the back of her head.

"It was really kind of neat," Loni explains. "He took little tiny plugs of hair and skin from the back of my head and transplanted them on the side. He'd put a plug, leave a space, put another plug, all over the area. After that healed and the transplants were doing well, he took more plugs from another section of my scalp and filled in the empty spaces."

Loni spent four days in the hospital and returned to school two weeks later wearing a big bandage on her head. "People who didn't know me thought I was trying to start a new fashion trend," she laughs. Today, Loni, 20, is busy getting on with her life. "My hair looks much the same as it did before the accident," she says. "I can style it any way I want. I'm growing it long, and I've had it permed and highlighted." Loni admits that memories of the accident come back, but, she says, "I haven't been traumatized by it. And I'm glad that facial plastic surgery gave me back a normal head."

and sometimes it skips a generation. It's entirely possible to have a bald father and bald uncles and enjoy a full head of hair all your life, if you inherited your hair genes from the other side of your family. On the other hand, if male relatives on both your mother's and your father's sides of your family started losing their hair in their early twenties and you are already noticing definite signs of a thinning hairline, you may well look the way they do by the time you reach your forties.

"Can anything be done about premature hair loss?"

There are several surgical techniques for treating male-pattern baldness. These are expensive and can involve a major investment of time, but are often sought after by men who aren't willing to accept baldness. The most common procedures are scalp flap surgery, punch grafts, and *scalp reduction surgery,* in which the facial plastic surgeon reduces the bald area by stretching hair-bearing scalp and cutting out the bald area.

But hair replacement surgery is not appropriate for a teenager who has just started to notice thinning hair. It is very important that the surgeon determine what the balding pattern is going to be. If the surgery is done too early, before the final balding pattern can be established, it can have very undesirable results. For example, a strip of hair-bearing scalp could end up in the middle of an area from which surrounding hair has receded.

"Hair loss is no big deal. I just noticed in the mirror this morning that my hairline is receding. It happens to everyone."

Hair loss certainly does happen to many men, and not all are bothered by it. Losing your hair doesn't mean losing your attractiveness. Many women find baldness sexy. It's all a matter of your attitude. If you are beginning to lose hair due to male-pattern baldness, try not to worry too much about it. If you find it really bothers you, you may want to look into possible surgical solutions when you reach your early thirties.

"I've heard there's a new drug you can rub on your head to stop baldness. What about it?"

The drug is called Rogaine® or minoxidil, and it does appear to cause hair growth in some people when applied to the scalp. At this point, doctors are not sure why it works, or even how well it works.

Head Lice Leaves Girl Bald

It was a long and painful route that led Rachel to a facial plastic surgeon. It began when she was seven years old. An epidemic of head lice ravaged her school, and, unfortunately, Rachel didn't escape the infestation. Her mother took her to her pediatrician, who prescribed a medicated shampoo.

Rachel vividly remembers what happened next. "My mom took the shampoo and began washing my hair at the kitchen sink. As she combed it out, my hair immediately began coming out in big clumps." Rachel returned to her doctor, but he was unable to determine what had gone wrong. Some of the hair grew back, but Rachel was left with a large permanent bald spot on the top of her head.

Although a number of treatments were tried, Rachel's case proved to be a stubborn one and the bald spot remained as she entered adolescence. The teasing from her classmates had ended by then and she had become expert at styling her hair to cover the bald area. Nonetheless, Rachel still felt self-conscious. She was careful to avoid swimming and activities that might reveal the bald area, and she dreaded the thought that a boyfriend might want to touch her hair.

Finally, Rachel learned of a facial plastic surgeon who had been successful in treating baldness. Despite her disappointment with other treatments, she decided to take another chance. At the consultation, the surgeon assured Rachel that he could help her. The solution to her problem was to be a technique called tissue expansion.

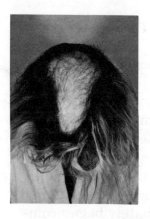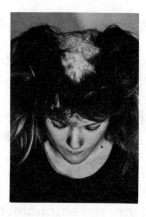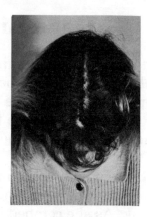

The series of photos above show the success of Rachel's tissue expansion surgery. At left her head is tilted to show the area of hair loss. The center photo shows the tissue expanders in place with hair styling to minimize the effect. Finally, the photo at right shows the small scar that is all that remains.

Balloons were implanted on either side of Rachel's head above her ears, and her mother learned to inject them with sterile water. By the second week bulges were appearing, but Rachel had no trouble covering them. "I bought myself six or seven hats and just went wherever I wanted to," she recalls. "After that many years of dealing with this problem, I knew how to make my hair look good!" After six or seven weeks of tissue expansion, Rachel had the surgery. "He just took the balloons out and closed it up," she explains. "The surgery was not painful—of course, I was asleep. I took pain killers for a day or two afterward."

Now Rachel is growing her hair long—something she hasn't been able to do for years. The bald spot is gone, and all that remains is a scar just slightly wider than a normal part.

Although it has caused hair growth in some people, in some of those cases the "hair" was nothing more than fuzz. It seems to work best right on the crown of the head, and it rarely has any effect around the hairline or at the temples.

Some researchers feel that Rogaine® can slow down the progress of male-pattern baldness. For this reason, it may be useful for teens and other young men who are just beginning to lose their hair. But more studies are needed to find out whether its long-term effects are truly beneficial. Rogaine® does need some existing hair, at least "peach fuzz," to work. Thus, it often works better on females, as they don't usually bald completely. Rogaine® is an expensive treatment—a one-month supply can cost more than $45. And once you start using the drug, you must use it for life. If you stop using it, all new hair growth falls out within a few months. If you are interested in trying Rogaine®, consult a dermatologist or a facial plastic surgeon regarding its use.

Hair Loss Because of Disease

"What can cause someone's hair to just start falling out? This is happening to my girlfriend and she's really worried about it."

Hair grows in cycles, and losing up to a hundred hairs a day can be normal. But if you are treating your hair right, and it is still falling out in large enough amounts to cause noticeable thinning, you may have a problem that should be checked out. Abnormal hair loss is rare in young people, but it can happen. It may be brought on by extreme stress or illness, but it is more likely to be the result of an immunological disorder known as alopecia areata.

There are three types of alopecia areata: The *areata* type means bald spots within hairy parts of head, *totalis* is total hair loss on the head, and *universalis* is total hair loss on all parts of the body.

What happens, simply, is that the person's immune system attacks the hair follicles as though they were foreign bodies, causing the hair to fall out. Unfortunately there is no type of facial plastic surgery that can help this kind of hair loss. If you do have a problem with abnormal hair loss, consult your dermatologist. Topical prescription medicine may help restore the lost hair. Perhaps your hair loss is only temporary.

What about Too Much Hair?

"I hate seeing facial hair on girls," comments Braden, 16. "Why do some girls have it, and what can they do about it?"

Seventeen-year-old Nick agrees that facial hair on girls is a turnoff. "One of the nicest girls I know has hair growing on her face. How can she get rid of it?"

Excess facial hair on girls may indicate a hormone imbalance. Thus, seeing your dermatologist or family doctor should be your first step. If the hair growth is caused by a medical problem, solving the problem may eliminate the hair. The cause may be genetic or both children and adults may grow excess facial hair as a result of a metabolic disorder. Girls also sometimes develop excess hair as result of birth control pills, which contain male hormones.

If you have no underlying medical problem, you can bleach the hair to camouflage it, or you can remove it temporarily by shaving, tweezing, or using a *depilatory* (over-the-counter hair remover). The only permanent way to remove unwanted hair is by electrolysis. This involves using a fine electric needle to destroy the individual hair-producing follicles. Electrolysis is done in some beauty salons, but if you decide to have this done, you may prefer to get a recommendation from your dermatologist or family doctor. Electrolysis is also done by dermatologists and professional technicians working with some facial plastic surgeons.

V

Finding Good Healthcare

15

Don't Expect Miracles

"Cindy Crawford—now there's a model I'd like to look like. She's just perfect with her beautiful eyes and sultry appearance," comments Jodi, 17.

"Can you believe how sexy looking Patrick Swayze is? His eyes and his jaw are just perfect," enthuses Marti, 14.

Ah, perfection! Do you ever wish you could look perfect? Everyone feels this way at times. But most people realize, down deep, that looking "perfect" is not the answer to everything. If you have a problem with your face, facial plastic surgery may help you look better. But it is not the road to perfection. Facial plastic surgery can help refine your facial features, but it cannot make you beautiful or change your outlook and personality. In fact, people who expect facial plastic surgery to make them perfect should not have surgery at all.

If you are considering facial plastic surgery, your first step should be to think seriously about your own motivations. One of the first questions the surgeon will ask you is, "Why do you want to have facial plastic surgery?"

The doctor may interview you at length, ask you to complete a detailed evaluation form, or send you for an assessment by a psychologist. You may be asked questions that seem irrelevant to you, but they are important for your surgeon, who needs to weed out patients who are expecting miracles that surgery cannot deliver. It is important that you want the surgery for yourself. If you are at the surgeon's office because you think your parents are disappointed with your appearance or your boyfriend or girlfriend thinks you ought to do something about your nose, it's better to wait. After all, this is your face. If you have surgery for the wrong reasons, you may end up feeling guilty or angry after you go through with it.

"What kind of people have surgery like this? No one I know ever did," comments Matt, 15, who is from a small town in Oklahoma.

Years ago, the only people who had facial plastic surgery were movie stars and wealthy socialites. In fact, some people used to think anyone who had facial plastic surgery was neurotic or emotionally disturbed. Even some psychologists shared this view. Today, attitudes have changed. Movie stars still have facial plastic surgery, of course, but the majority of people seeking facial plastic surgery today are ordinary people who basically like themselves. Most choose facial plastic surgery because they are bothered by a facial feature that is out of balance with the rest of their face. They are not trying to be perfect; they just want to improve a specific feature and, thus, feel better about the way they look.

Is Facial Plastic Surgery Right for You?
A Self-evaluation Test to Help You Decide

Here are some questions to think about before you visit a facial plastic surgeon. They are very similar to some of the questions the doctor may ask.

General Questions
1. Exactly what features do I want changed?
2. How long have I been thinking about having surgery?
3. What caused me to begin thinking about it?
4. Do I feel guilty or embarrassed about having facial plastic surgery?
5. How do my parents feel about my decision?

Medical Questions
1. Have I ever had any unusual bleeding or poor scarring?
2. Have I ever had recurrent nosebleeds?
3. Do I bruise more easily than most people?
4. Am I on any sort of special diet?
5. Do I have asthma or any chronic lung condition?
6. Do I smoke or use drugs?

Personality Questions
1. Does life often seem like a burden to me?
2. Am I pessimistic about the future?
3. Has there been any recent emotional crisis in my life?
4. Am I considered introverted or unusually quiet and shy?
5. Am I overly sensitive to the opinions of others?

"I heard of someone who wanted a nose job, but the surgeon said no. Why would a doctor do that?"

Facial plastic surgeons try to assess the level of self-esteem a patient has and whether the surgery is being sought for an appropriate reason. Sometimes people go to facial plastic surgeons hoping to solve psychological or personal problems. This is never a good reason for having facial plastic surgery. Surgeons may say no if you have an inappropriate reason for wanting the surgery or seem out of touch with reality, if it seems you are being pressured by someone else to have surgery, or if you want something that realistically cannot be done through surgery.

"How long do these surgical changes last? Are they good for just a few months and then everything returns to the way it was?"

Surgery is forever. That is why it is so important to be sure that surgery is really right for you. It's not like a beauty makeover that can be washed off if you don't like it. Facial plastic surgery is basically a permanent change.

"Can a facial plastic surgeon take truly ugly people and make them look beautiful or even moderately cute?"

Facial plastic surgery techniques can only refine and enhance the features that a person already has. Those old spy stories about someone getting a whole new identity by dyeing his hair and getting facial plastic surgery are just fiction. Facial plastic surgery cannot give anyone a whole new face. And remember, true beauty also takes into account a person's personality, attitude, poise, and the way he or she acts.

16

Talk to Your Parents

"I'd get a big lecture if I asked for facial plastic surgery. My parents would say it was the 'principle' of the whole thing and that I should be glad I'm healthy and have a normal face," is 14-year-old Kevin's response to how his parents would react if he asked for facial plastic surgery.

Megan, 16, believes her parents would be a little more understanding. "They would talk to me for a long time about it and try to convince me that it wasn't necessary, but they would probably say okay if they realized how serious I was. They might make me pay for it, though."

"My mother and aunt both have had rhinoplasties, so I think they would be understanding," comments Angie, 17. "My dad would think it was ridiculous and too expensive."

Even before you talk to a surgeon about having facial plastic surgery, you should bring up the subject with your parents. For some young people, that hurdle may seem more intimidating than the surgery itself.

Often parents react negatively at first to the idea of facial plastic surgery for their children, even if those children are grown. It is a major decision, after all, and not one that can be reversed if you change your mind after the surgery is done. Moreover, parents tend to see their children as just fine the way they are, or likely to "grow out" of any awkwardness in looks or behavior. But you will never know how your parents will react until you broach the subject with them.

Perhaps they will feel that your big nose is a precious heritage from granddad or dear old Aunt Sophie. But it's just as likely that they always have been aware of your ill-fitting facial feature but hesitated to say anything about it. They may have been afraid of making you feel bad or unloved. Or maybe they are just waiting until you are old enough to have surgery or until you express an interest in it yourself.

Most parents really do have their children's best interests at heart. It may help to share your feelings with your family doctor, school counselor, clergyman, or an adult friend whom your parents trust. If you are truly a good candidate for surgery, it is quite possible that your parents will agree once they understand how important it is to you. Don't be discouraged if they continue to ignore your concerns. Try to understand *their* concerns. Listen to what they have to say. And try to get them to listen, read, or talk to experts in the field in order to increase their understanding of the subject.

Facial plastic surgeons report that parents often go through four stages in their efforts to deal with a child's desire for facial plastic surgery. The first is denial, or an unwillingness to accept that their child is less than perfect. The second stage often is anger. The parents may feel the child is badgering them with his persistence. A form of bargaining may follow. For example, the parents may say something like, "Forget about the nose, and I'll let you go on a ski trip." There may be depression on the part of the parents, who frequently feel they have failed their child in some way.

Finally there is acceptance, when the parents recognize that this is a very important step in a young person's life and not only agree to the surgery but give their full support as well.

"Do my parents have to see the doctor with me? There are some things that I just can't say in front of them."

At least one parent should accompany you to the initial consultation. This tells the doctor that you are really serious about surgery and that your parents are willing to consider it. A minor must have parental permission for something this serious, and a young adult may psychologically need that parental nod of approval.

An understanding surgeon can help if there are things you don't feel comfortable saying in front of your parents. One physician felt that a girl who had come in for nose surgery was holding something back. He told her parents he needed to see her again, this time by herself. The girl's parents agreed. When the girl came in alone, she admitted that she hesitated to have surgery because she feared hurting her father. Her large, hooked nose was identical to his, and he seemed happy enough with it. The surgeon explained that a nose that looks perfectly okay on a man may be unattractive on a woman. With the girl's permission, he let the father know of her concerns about hurting him, and the father was able to reassure his daughter of his support for her decision.

"How old must you be to have facial surgery?"

"Is there a best age to have facial plastic surgery?"

Most facial plastic surgery procedures cannot be done until your bone structure has completed its growth. This usually means about 15 or 16 for girls and 16 or 17 for boys, but can vary according to the individual. Some girls have achieved their full growth and facial development by age 13 or 14. Your facial plastic surgeon will be able to determine if you are old enough for the procedure you desire.

One exception is otoplasty, the operation to correct deformed or fly-away ears, which can be done on patients as young as six or seven. Removal of port wine stains and scar revision also can be done at early ages, and removal of certain moles and birthmarks is recommended before puberty since that's when they are most likely to become cancerous.

There is really no "best" age. Young people tend to heal rather quickly, but there is nothing wrong with waiting until you are in your early twenties or older. Your facial features will change and mature somewhat as you do, so a problem that seems overwhelming when you are 16—say, "chipmunk cheeks"—could disappear altogether before your late twenties.

17

Choose a Specialist Who Cares

"Suppose I do decide to have facial plastic surgery. How would I find the best surgeon?" asks Melanie, 16.

"I wouldn't know how to judge whether a surgeon was good or not," adds Tracey, 17. "My face is pretty important to me, and I would be devastated if it didn't come out right."

If you are seriously considering facial plastic surgery, you will want to find a surgeon who specializes in the procedure(s) you're contemplating. You'll not want to trust your face to anyone but a facial plastic surgeon who has established a reputation for achieving good results.

Such a surgeon will be skilled at handling all of the unique conditions that may arise. This is important because surgery is not an exact, predictable science. Individual results always are affected by

such factors as age, overall health, skin texture, bone structure,
ability to heal, and the nature of the problem.

Here are some tips for finding a facial plastic surgeon:

- First, talk to your parents.

- Talk to people who have had facial plastic surgery as well
  as their families and friends.

- Ask your family doctor or other medical practitioner whom
  you trust.

- Check the *Directory of Medical Specialists* at your local
  library.

- Call the referral service of your county medical society and
  ask for the names of surgeons who limit their practice to
  the face.

- Call the toll-free number of the Facial Plastic Surgery Information Service.

    In the U.S.: (800) 332-FACE
    In Canada: (800) 523-FACE

  You will receive a list of board-certified surgeons in your
  immediate geographic area.

- Look through the Yellow Pages and other advertisements.
  Not all doctors advertise, but many see it as a good way to
  introduce their services to the community. But beware of a
  hard sell. Don't try to find a facial plastic surgeon in the
  same way you'd look for a used car dealership.

"Do facial plastic surgeons have any special credentials?"

They do indeed, and you should feel free to ask what credentials a surgeon has when you make your appointment or at the initial consultation. You will learn that a great deal of training and experience lie behind any facial plastic surgeon's reputation for consistently good results with the procedure you want.

Typically, a facial plastic surgeon will have attended four years of college and four years of medical school, and taken a residency of five or six years. Many also have taken a fellowship in facial plastic surgery, a year of advanced study with a senior surgeon. Most continue their education through courses of study given by their medical specialty society.

At some point during training, medical students choose a field in which to specialize and later are examined by a medical specialty board. Several boards certify facial plastic surgeons. The largest number of facial plastic surgeons are *otolaryngologist-head and neck surgeons*, whose special training in the complex head and neck area gives them thorough knowledge of both functional and aesthetic or cosmetic repairs. Other surgeons who perform facial plastic surgery procedures are boarded as general plastic surgeons. Their training includes the whole body, and they are as likely to specialize in, say, hand surgery as facial surgery. Also, dermatologists perform some facial plastic surgery procedures, specifically those that affect the skin. Ophthalmologists sometimes perform facial plastic surgery procedures that involve the soft tissue around the eye.

Again, the most important questions to ask are how frequently the surgeon performs the surgery you want and whether his results are consistently good.

"How can you tell if a particular surgeon is right for you?"

Once you have narrowed your choices to one or two highly recommended facial plastic surgeons, you should make an appointment for a consultation. Your first impression will tell you a lot. Does the doctor seem comfortable dealing with young people? Do you feel that you are treated like a person, or does the doctor talk over your head and address all of his or her comments to your parents? Are all your questions answered thoroughly? Does the doctor take time with you, or are you made to feel rushed?

Here are some questions that you and your parents might want to ask the surgeon before you make the final decision:

- How many patients my age have you treated?

- How often do you do this procedure (nasal surgery, scar removal, or whatever you are interested in) each year?

- Can you show me "before" and "after" pictures of some of your patients who have had this kind of surgery? (Note: Some facial plastic surgeons, in maintaining their patients' confidentiality, do not show photos of other patients.)

- Do you have any patients my age who would be willing to talk to me about their surgery?

If you have any feeling of discomfort with the first surgeon you see, don't hesitate to visit a second one. It is important for you to feel comfortable with your surgeon (and he or she with you).

18

Pre-op Jitters
and Post-op Care

"I would be so afraid to have surgery," declares Molly, 16. "I'm afraid my face would be swollen afterward, and I would feel self-conscious. What if the doctor didn't do it right and I could never go back to the way I used to look? Plus, the pain—I know I couldn't stand it."

On the other hand, Nan, also 16, says, "I would love to have something done to my nose, but my parents say it's too expensive."

Andrea, 14, remembers being very anxious when she went for her rhinoplasty. "I wasn't afraid of the surgery or the pain, but I worried about whether I was being too vain or frivolous."

"Being put to sleep for an operation is what scares me," confides Marc, 19. "You have absolutely no control."

It's natural to be nervous about something as serious as facial plastic surgery. After all, having surgery is not an everyday occurrence. But if you are serious about having a facial feature corrected, it may help to know that many teens just like you have had facial plastic surgery and felt good about the results.

If you do have concerns, talk to your surgeon. He or she may put you in touch with other young people who have had similar surgery. Talking to someone who has been through it can help. Be sure you get all your questions answered before you actually go in for surgery.

Fears about Risks Usually Are Unwarranted

"Will the change look natural? I don't want to look like I've just had something done."

There is nothing "plastic" about facial plastic surgery. Your improved appearance should appear perfectly natural. In fact, close friends may not even realize exactly what is different about you unless you tell them. Often people will comment that a person who has just had facial plastic surgery looks "rested" or "prettier" or "healthy," not realizing that there has been a surgical change.

"Are there a lot of scars after surgery?"

For most procedures, incisions are small and hidden and aren't noticeable once healed. The exception is for patients who have a tendency to develop keloids (see chapter 12). If you have ever had difficulty with wounds healing in the past, be sure to let your surgeon know before the surgery is performed.

"How long does the surgery take?"

It depends on the procedure. A simple chin implant can be accomplished in less than an hour. Orthognathic surgery on the jaw may take several hours. Most procedures take between one and three hours. Many procedures are performed in the surgeon's office or ambulatory care facility. Other surgeons—and patients—prefer a hospital setting. Be sure to discuss your feelings on this issue with your surgeon. And make sure your surgeon has hospital privileges in case you need emergency care.

"Will I have to be put to sleep?"

It depends. Often a mild anesthetic is injected into the area where the surgery is to be performed and you are given intravenous anesthesia, eliminating the need for being put to sleep entirely and allowing you to return home that same day. If you or your surgeon opt for general anesthesia, an overnight hospital stay may be required.

"Will I look grotesque once the surgery is over?"

Certainly not grotesque, although there will be evidence of surgery having been performed. To learn how specific features heal, read the earlier chapter on the procedure you want.

"Can facial plastic surgery affect the other features of the face?"

"Can facial plastic surgery damage nerves and blood vessels?"

Complications are rare in facial plastic surgery, but remember that no surgery is completely risk-free. Your surgeon will explain any possible risks associated with the procedure you are considering. But be aware that surgery is a two-way proposition. It is vitally important that you follow the instructions of your surgeon to the

Patient Rights, Responsibilities

Proper patient care begins with consideration of the patient's rights and responsibilities. Facial plastic surgeons strive to treat their patients with respect, consideration, and dignity. Some surgeons have even gone so far as to document what their patients can expect in a "Patient Bill of Rights." Such a bill of rights might include the following:

The Patient's Rights

As a patient, you have a right to:

- Receive kind and respectful care.

- Have knowledge of the name of the physician who has primary responsibility for coordinating your care and the names and professional relationships of other physicians who will see you.

- Receive information from your physician about your problem, your course of treatment, and prospects for recovery in terms you can understand.

- Participate actively in decisions regarding your medical care. To the extent permitted by law, this includes the right to refuse treatment.

- Receive full consideration of privacy concerning your medical care program. This includes confidential treatment of all communications and records pertaining to your care.

- Be informed by your surgeon of continuing healthcare requirements following treatment.

- Examine and receive an explanation of your bill regardless of source of payment.

The Other Side of the Coin

Of course, patients who are treated fairly and responsibly must reciprocate in turn. As a patient, you have certain responsibilities that, if heeded, will enable your surgeon to handle your care more effectively and safely.

These responsibilities include filling out all questionnaires to the best of your knowledge and being honest with the surgeon and staff about your own health problems. For instance, bleeding disorders, heart disease, and personal habits, such as smoking and heavy use of alcohol or drugs, could have adverse effects on your surgical results. It is imperative that your facial plastic surgeon know of them. You also must tell your surgeon about any prescription or over-the-counter drugs you are taking, because they may affect your surgeon's choice of anesthesia, pain medication, etc. This information is vitally important and will be kept strictly confidential.

It is also vitally important that you follow your surgeon's instructions to the letter, both pre- and post-operatively, and that you ask for further explanation of any instructions or comments that you do not understand. Any surgical procedure involves some risk, such as bleeding, infection, or reaction to anesthesia. Omitting facts about health problems could endanger your health or leave you with less-than-optimum results.

letter for the best results. Fears about surgery often are expressed, but they usually are unwarranted. Hundreds of thousands of people of all ages successfully undergo facial plastic surgery each year. Your surgeon should be able to reassure you if you have any concerns.

Pain Is Rarely a Major Problem

"How much does facial plastic surgery hurt?"

"Is medication required after surgery?"

Surgery does involve a certain degree of discomfort for most people, but the majority of people who have had these procedures describe the pain as "mild" or "moderate." Some report no real pain at all. The surgery itself should be nearly painless. If you have discomfort during the healing period, your surgeon will prescribe pain medication.

Costs of Facial Plastic Surgery Vary

"How much does facial plastic surgery cost?"

"I'd like to have surgery, but we probably couldn't afford it."

It's true: Facial plastic surgery—like any surgery—is somewhat expensive. Depending on the complexity of the procedure, costs can vary from five hundred to several thousand dollars. Costs for specific procedures also vary from one surgeon to the next and among different parts of the country.

"Does insurance pay the bill like it does for other operations?"

Facial plastic surgical procedures that are intended just to improve your appearance usually are not covered by insurance. If you have

The Costs of Facial Plastic Surgery

Surgeons vary widely in the fees they charge for facial plastic surgery procedures. Under the law, surgeons set their own fees: Your facial plastic surgeon will inform you of the costs at your initial consultation. As a generalized guide, however, here are some price ranges, which do not include the costs of the hospital, anesthesia, nursing care, and medication:

Ears (both)	$1,000—$4,500
Chin implant	$ 500—$2,000
Nose	$1,500—$6,000
Dermabrasion (full face)	$1,000—$3,500
Collagen injections (per visit)	$ 200—$ 350
Scalp reduction	$1,000—$3,500
Two eyelids (upper or lower)	$1,000—$4,000

a medical problem that will be repaired by the surgery, then insurance usually pays at least part of the cost. For example, orthognathic surgery to correct the alignment of the jaw is often covered by insurance. Nose surgery that repairs breathing problems should be partially covered. It's wise to check with your insurance company before scheduling facial plastic surgery.

Once the Surgery Is Done
"How soon after surgery can I wear makeup?"

If you have had dermabrasion, you must wait about ten days to two weeks before applying makeup. For most other procedures, waiting is not necessary. Just don't put makeup over any incisions until they are healed—usually in about a week. Ask your surgeon for additional instructions.

"How long does it take before you are able to get back into your normal routine after facial plastic surgery?"

Most people can go back to school or work about a week after facial plastic surgery. Bandages and stitches are usually removed by that time, and you should be feeling back to normal. Often young people schedule surgery during a holiday period, say Christmas or spring break, so they won't have to miss school.

You will have to avoid activities that may strain the area that was operated on. If you had nose surgery, for example, you will have to be careful not to let anything hit your nose for at least six weeks.

Most surgeons recommend that you avoid athletic activities for a while. If you swim or dive, your surgeon may advise you to give up this sport for a month or two. Contact sports and very strenuous workouts usually are ruled out for about six weeks. Your surgeon will give you specific information.

"Can I go out in the sun after my surgery?"

Skin that has been operated on is particularly sensitive following surgery, and you can get a severe burn without realizing it. Your surgeon may recommend that you avoid excessive exposure to the sun for several weeks after surgery. It is often advised that patients not schedule surgery too soon before a ski vacation or trip to the beach.

19

Put Your Best Face Forward

"I've had my surgery, and my incisions have begun to heal," says Kathy, 19. "I can't wait to go out and see how people react. But I'm a little scared, too. What happens now?"

First of all, after surgery give yourself time to heal. You may feel unusually wiped out for a day or two, or even a little depressed. Fatigue is natural—after all, you *have* had surgery. Take it easy, and it will pass in a day or two.

If you find yourself feeling depressed, remember that the final results are not yet visible. The scars will heal and shrink, the swelling will go down, and the discoloration will go away. As time passes, your face will only get better.

"Will people look at me and say I look good after surgery?"

They may. But don't be surprised if they don't even notice anything different. They may notice that you look great but not really know why (unless you have told them about your surgery).

If you do want to keep your surgery a secret, here are some tips that may help:

- Just before you go in for surgery, make some other change in your appearance. Get a dramatically different haircut, change your hairstyle to something curlier or straighter, or use clips or combs in a new way. People will notice the obvious difference and not focus so much on the surgical change.
- Draw attention away from your face. Try an eye-catching bracelet, a wild belt, a big pin or button, a scarf, or some other accessory to attract attention downward. Or wear a great new hat to encourage people to look upward.
- Keep your makeup simple and just concentrate on concealing bruises until your face is completely healed. Avoid anything that draws attention to the incision scars. For example, don't wear a turtleneck right after chin surgery or dramatic eye colors if you just had your eyes done.

"Do people feel more normal or better-looking after having surgery?"

Correcting an obvious facial problem through facial plastic surgery usually makes people feel more confident in themselves. You will still look like yourself—you will just look a little better without that feature that has always bothered you.

Remember, having facial plastic surgery is something you do for *you!* Don't expect others to treat you differently or see you as more attractive. Just relax and enjoy your new appearance!

Glossary

Alopecia areata—An immunological disorder causing hair loss.

Ambulatory care facility—A facility for same-day surgery at a hospital, clinic, or doctor's office.

Augmentation mentoplasty—An operation to enlarge the chin using artificial implants or bone grafts.

Blepharoplasty—The removal of excess fat or skin from the upper or lower eyelids.

Cannula—A narrow tube, no larger than a soda straw, used in liposuction.

Chemical peel—Use of a diluted acid on the face, which causes the top layers of skin to slough off, leaving smoother, more youthful-looking skin.

Collagen—A natural protein substance that can be injected to fill pock marks, wrinkles, or other skin indectations.

Comedo—A blackhead.

Computer-assisted imaging—A new technology that enables a facial plastic surgeon to predict surgical results and "age" your face with a high degree of accuracy.

Contracted scar—A scar that tightened while healing, pulling facial features out of place.

Depilatory—A product to remove unwanted hair from the body.

Dermabrasion—Facial sanding or the use of an abrasive material to buff off the top layers of skin, often used in removing acne scars.

Electrolysis—A procedure in which unwanted hairs are removed permanently.

Elliptical excision—A procedure for removing moles.

Facial plastic surgeon—A surgeon who specializes in cosmetic and reconstructive surgery of the head and neck. The facial plastic surgeon may be boarded by the American Board of Otolaryngology, the American Board of Plastic Surgery, the American Board of Ophthalmology, or the American Board of Dermatology.

Geometric broken line closure—A surgical procedure to break up a straight scar by cutting geometric shapes into the scar tissue.

Injectable fillers—Material injected into the skin to "plump up" specific areas, such as acne scars. See *collagen*.

Keloid scars—Thick, irregularly shaped scars with a raised appearance caused by the abnormal growth of fibrous tissue.

Lasers—Intense beams of light used to painlessly "burn away" moles and marks caused by enlarged blood vessels and broken capillaries under the skin.

Liposuction—The removal of excess fat cells by suction.

Malar augmentation—Cheek implants.

Male-pattern baldness—Hereditary baldness common in men.

Melanin—Brownish pigment that determines skin color.

Melanoma—A cancerous tumor.

Miniplates—Small, thin strips of metal used to hold fractured bones together after an accident.

Nasal septum—The internal wall of the nose.

Orthognathic surgery—A surgical procedure to reposition or realign bones of the upper and lower jaw.

Otolaryngologist-head and neck surgeon—A surgeon who specializes in treating the complex head and neck area and is boarded by the American Board of Otolaryngology.

Otoplasty—A surgical procedure to reshape cartilage of protruding ears.

Port wine stain—A purplish colored birthmark resulting from enlarged blood vessels in the skin.

Ptosis surgery—Surgery that corrects droopy eyelids.

Punch elevation—A process of cutting into deep scars to raise the level of the skin.

Punch graft—A type of hair transplant.

Rhinoplasty—A procedure to change the width, size, and/or shape of the nose.

Scalp flaps—A repositioning of hair-bearing skin to treat baldness.

Scalp reduction—A surgical procedure to reduce bald areas of the scalp.

Scar revision—A surgical procedure to camouflage a scar.

Sebaceous glands—Glands in the skin that produce oil.

Septorhinoplasty—A procedure to correct breathing problems by removing blockages in the nasal passages.

Serial excision—A series of procedures in which a scar is excised a bit at a time.

Skin flaps—A repositioning of uninjured "donor" skin to cover adjacent injuries without separating donor skin from its blood supply.

Tangential excision—A procedure to remove moles by shaving the mole flat with the surface of the skin.

Tissue expansion—A technique to stretch healthy skin, usually by implanting small expanders (balloons) under the skin, for skin flap reconstruction.

W-plasty—A surgical procedure to break up a straight scar by cutting a row of tiny W or Z shapes into the scar tissue.

Z-plasty—A surgical procedure to elongate a scar so it does not contract surrounding skin.

About the American Academy of Facial Plastic and Reconstructive Surgery

The American Academy of Facial Plastic and Reconstructive Surgery (AAFPRS), an international medical society of more than 3,200 facial plastic surgeons, is the largest association of facial plastic surgeons in the world. Membership is open to otolaryngologist-head and neck surgeons, dermatologists, ophthalmologists, general plastic surgeons, and other surgeons who are certified by an American examining board of specialists or its equivalent, and have training or experience in facial plastic surgery.

In addition to being board-certified, Academy fellows must be board-certified fellows of the American College of Surgeons or its equivalent, and citizens or residents of the United States or Canada. They must have been actively engaged in practicing facial plastic surgery for a period of three years prior to application, and they must submit a detailed report of 35 major facial plastic and reconstructive surgical procedures performed within a 12-month period.

The AAFPRS promotes the study, research, and scientific advancement of facial plastic surgery and all related basic sciences. Members are devoted to expanding the knowledge and improving the skills of facial plastic surgeons and training residents and other young physicians interested in the specialty.

The AAFPRS's program of continuing medical education is widely respected by the medical community. Since it was established in 1964, the AAFPRS has been and is dedicated to the dissemination of knowledge. The program of courses offered annually by the Academy includes more than 35 seminars and workshops on all major aspects of facial plastic surgery. Its graduate fellowship program represents one of the finest opportunities for the education of facial plastic surgeons in the nation. Two programs—the observational education program and the visiting professors program—give members the opportunity to observe selected senior Academy fellows in their own operating rooms and offices, and senior members to share their knowledge with residents in university hospital settings. In addition, an outstanding videotape series gives all members the opportunity to view the techniques of senior members. An awards program each year recognizes clinical or research-oriented contributions to the field. Several research grants are made each year.

SUPPLEMENTAL INFORMATION

A series of brochures, a newsletter, and a book on facial plastic surgery procedures not covered in this book are available from the Facial Plastic Surgery Information Service, Inc., which also will tell you the names of facial plastic surgeons in your area. Contact FPSIS at 1101 Vermont Ave. NW, Suite 404, Washington, DC 20005; or call (800) 332-FACE in the U.S. and (800) 523-FACE in Canada.

Acknowledgments

The publication of *The Teen Face Book: A Question and Answer Guide to Skin Care, Cosmetics, and Facial Plastic Surgery* seems especially appropriate this year, as 1989 marks the 25th anniversary of the founding of the American Academy of Facial Plastic and Reconstructive Surgery—the largest association of facial plastic surgeons in the world.

Since its inception, education has been the primary goal of this Academy. Whereas early educational programs aimed at providing members with continuing medical education, in recent years the Academy's efforts have been extended to include public education about the rapidly advancing specialty of facial plastic surgery.

The Academy's first book—*The Face Book: The Pros and Cons of Facial Plastic Surgery*, written primarily for adults—was cited by *U.S. News and World Report* as "among the best" of a handful of books for the lay public. Its sequel, *The Teen Face Book: A Question and Answer Guide to Skin Care, Cosmetics, and Facial Plastic Surgery*, seeks to be equally valuable to teens and young adults. It is not a book that advocates facial plastic surgery, but rather one that frankly discusses how to look your best through a variety of means, thereby improving your self-confidence.

The information contained herein represents the cumulative knowledge and experience of all Academy members during the past 25 years. Their contributions to the field have been reviewed for this book by a 10-member editorial board, chaired by Norman J. Pastorek, M.D., with members including: Ferdinand F. Becker, Jr., M.D.; Ted A. Cook, M.D.; Peter M. Goldman, M.D.; Jeffrey N. Hausfeld, M.D.; Richard G. Holt, M.D.; Devinder S. Mangat, M.D.; Louie L. Patseavouras, M.D.; Stephen W. Perkins, M.D.; and Dale H. Rice, M.D.

Also contributing to individual chapters were: G. Jan Beekhuis, M.D.; Edwin A. Cortez, M.D.; Steven M. Denenberg, M.D.; Richard W. Fleming, M.D.; Richard E. Hayden, M.D.; Sheldon S. Kabaker, M.D.; Frank M.

Kamer, M.D.; Frank C. Koranda, M.D.; John A. McCurdy, Jr., M.D.; Daniel E. Rousso, M.D.; David M. Sarver, D.M.D.; Larry D. Schoenrock, M.D.; Robert L. Simons, M.D.; J. Regan Thomas, M.D.; and Paul H. Toffel, M.D.

It is a testament to these contributors' work that their patients so willingly granted permission to share their stories and photographs through this book. All names have been changed to protect patient confidentiality, but the cases are real and, the Academy believes, accurately reflect typical experiences.

Besides the debt of gratitude owed these facial plastic surgeons and their patients, the Academy would like to thank Paul Forbes and his associates at the Forbes Group and AAFPRS attorney Thomas Rhodes for their contributions.

Finally, for their work "in the trenches," pulling together the manuscript and gathering the art, we acknowledge the editorial team at the Business Service Network, especially Manager Susan Hill Rozynek; Senior Editor Debbie Demmon-Berger; Associate Editors Angela Martin, Fran Cohen Wickham, and Sharon Cool; Senior Designer Tamara Strickhouser; and Research Assistants Debbie Kallgren and Marcia A. Metzgar. This group interviewed more than 200 teens and young adults, from the metropolitan areas around New York City and Washington, D.C., to the heartlands of Kansas, to learn what role appearance plays in the lives of young people today—and what questions they would like answered, by the experts, about enhancing their own best features.

We hope this book gives young readers—and their parents—some insight into our members' untiring dedication to providing people of all ages with the highest quality possible of facial plastic surgery. If you are interested in learning more about facial plastic surgery or receiving the names of AAFPRS fellows in your area who participate in the Facial Plastic Surgery Information Service, please feel free to call (800) 332-FACE in the U.S. or (800) 523-FACE in Canada.

Lee VanBremen, Ph.D.
Executive Vice President, AAFPRS

Art Credits

Facial Plastic Surgery for Teens: A Parent's Guide

Should teens have facial plastic surgery?

Teenagers have many of the same concerns about their appearance that adults have. In fact, during adolescence, these concerns may be especially acute.

Parents sometimes worry that young people are overly preoccupied with their looks. As an adult, you are well aware that many of these fears and concerns will fade with time. Naturally, you don't want your child to do something irrevocable that may be regretted later.

But if your child has a serious need to change a particular feature; minimize skin blemishes, scars, or birthmarks; or address facial anomalies resulting from injury or disease, you should know that facial plastic surgery might be a valid option.

Common Procedures For Teenagers

These are the most common facial plastic surgery procedures done on teenagers:

Rhinoplasty—improves the size and shape of the nose to bring it into harmony with the rest of the face. It is done by removing excess bone and cartilage and sculpting the remaining structures. Breathing problems may be corrected in a combined procedure called *septorhinoplasty*.

Orthognathic Surgery—often performed on young people who have severe problems with their "bite" or jaw alignment. It may involve cooperation among the child's dentist, orthodontist, and oral or maxillofacial surgeon and is usually considered functional, rather than cosmetic, surgery.

Mentoplasty (chin augmentation)—correction for a receding chin by inserting a small plastic implant. The procedure often is done in conjunction with nasal plastic surgery, and may be combined with liposuction or lipectomy procedures for removing excess fat deposits from beneath the chin.

Otoplasty—the procedure for "pinning back' protruding ears or correcting ear deformities. This surgery can be done as early as age five or six.

Dermabrasion—a facial sanding procedure that is used to diminish severe acne and other scars.

Blepharoplasty—eyelid surgery for people of all ages who have unusually droopy, closed, or angry-looking eyes.

Reconstructive Surgery—a variety of techniques that includes bone grafts and implants, skin flaps and grafts, tissue expansion, scalp flap surgery, and other procedures that are used to correct congenital deformities and facial trauma. Young people who suffer serious injury in an automobile accident or on a motorcycle, bike, or skateboard; sports injuries or falls; burns; hair loss; attacks by humans or animals; or other facial injuries often can benefit from reconstructive facial plastic surgery procedures.

Scar Revision Surgery—to minimize visible facial scars that will not improve with time.

Birthmark Removal—Laser surgery and other techniques to remove unsightly birthmarks, including port wine stains.

Keep the Lines of Communication Open

The teen years are a time of change as young people work at developing a sense of physical self-image. They may experiment with new social roles as they try out various "looks."

During this time of life, more than at any other, self-esteem is closely linked with body image. Much anxiety can be generated by any defect or deformity, real or imagined. Young people tend to be self-conscious, and many teens go through periods when they wish they could change something about their face. This doesn't necessarily mean they should have facial plastic surgery, or even that they want to. But these concerns do deserve a sympathetic ear. As your teen matures, he or she will learn that no one is perfect and that perfection is no guarantee of success or happiness.

But what if your teenager does have a facial feature that truly disrupts facial harmony—such as a crooked nose, a receding chin, or protruding ears? First of all, don't emphasize the defect and be very careful before suggesting facial plastic surgery as a solution. Your teenager needs your approval to develop healthy self-esteem. The desire to change a facial defect must come from the individual, not family or friends.

If your child brings up the subject, listen and try to understand his or her concerns. Many young people hesitate to ask about facial plastic surgery, fearing parental disapproval. You may want to assure your child that you are willing to discuss possibilities. Talking about surgery doesn't mean a decision has been made.

Questions Parents Ask About Facial Plastic Surgery

How do I know the right time to take my child in for a consultation with a facial plastic surgeon?

The time to see a surgeon is when the child expresses serious concerns about a feature that may be corrected through facial plastic surgery. Don't pressure the child. The exceptions to this rule are if your child has protruding ears, a port wine stain, or other birth defects. Parents might encourage early consideration of correction for these problems to save their child a lifetime of teasing. Corrective procedures can be done effectively at a young age.

What if the child is not old enough for facial plastic surgery?

There is always benefit to learning how a problem will be affected by normal growth, and at what point surgical intervention might be helpful. An early consultation with a facial plastic surgeon will help you learn how to monitor growth and give you time to prepare for surgery if it is needed.

What is the right age for facial plastic surgery?

Protruding ears and some birth defects most frequently are correct-ed before a child starts school. If the child has a functional prob-lem—such as an underdeveloped lower jaw—see the doctor early to determine what the appropriate course of treatment should be. Other procedures are not done until the face has reached its full growth. This is usually 14 or 15 years of age for girls and 16 or 17 for boys.

What kind of people have facial plastic surgery? I don't want my child to be vain or preoccupied with perfection.

Teens who are seeking perfection or who wish to look like someone else—say a movie star or a particular model—are not considered good candidates for facial plastic surgery. Most people who have surgery are well adjusted individuals who basically like themselves but wish to change a feature with which they are dissatisfied.

How can I know whether surgery is right for my child?

The surgeon you consult will spend as much time as necessary to help you and your child make this decision. The child's emotional and physical well-being will be discussed as it relates to his or her being a good candidate for surgery.

Is there any way to predict how my child's features will change with maturity, or how my child will look after surgery?

Since healing differs with each individual, the surgeon cannot promise a specific result. However, facial plastic surgeons use sev-eral methods to show how a person's unique bone structure and covering tissues may react to surgery. These techniques—including sketching, use of mathematical measurements, and computer imaging—also may be used to demonstrate how a feature may change as the child matures.

Choosing a Surgeon

It is important to choose a surgeon with whom you and your child feel comfortable and confident. You may want to get a referral from your family doctor or ask friends and relatives who have had facial plastic surgery. Try to find a doctor who relates to teenagers, who listens well and takes plenty of time to answer any questions you or your teenager might have.

Be sure to look for a facial plastic surgeon who specializes in the particular procedure your child wants and who consistently gets good results.

Surgeons from many specialties have developed plastic surgery procedures. These specialties include otolaryngology–head and neck surgery, general surgery, dermatology, oral and maxillofacial surgery, ophthalmology, and neurosurgery. Consequently several specialties are qualified to perform plastic surgery.

Facial plastic surgeons specialize in performing cosmetic and reconstructive surgery on the face, head, and neck region. As a group, facial plastic surgeons, who, for the most part are board-certified in otolaryngology–head and neck surgery, do a major share of all facial plastic surgery performed in the United States. Because of their specialized training and in-depth knowledge about the face, head, and neck, these surgeons possess unique qualifications to provide patients with special insight and expertise into the conditions they treat.

The Initial Visit

During the initial visit, the surgeon will make a thorough evaluation of your child's problem, discuss possible treatment options, and talk about risks and cost. He will candidly answer all of your questions, so you can make a decision.

Pre-op and Post-op Considerations

Many facial plastic surgery procedures can be performed safely on an "outpatient" basis in an office surgery or an ambulatory surgery center. Some procedures may be done in a hospital, especially if the patient is very young or unusually nervous.

The Results to Expect

Facial plastic surgery cannot produce a miracle. Anyone who expects it to be the answer to personal problems is likely to be disappointed. Facial plastic surgery can minimize facial problems and improve appearance. The improvement, in turn, may enhance self-confidence. But surgery should not be expected to improve a teenager's social life or solve other problems.

The final results depend on the skill and experience of the surgeon, as well as the age, health, skin texture, bone structure, and healing capacity of the patient. A positive emotional attitude also is important. Young patients generally heal quickly and experience good results.

The Risks

The risks involved in most facial plastic surgery procedures are minimal. There are inherent risks in any surgical undertaking, of course, and these should be discussed thoroughly with your facial plastic surgeon. Many thousands of these procedures are performed successfully on young people each year.

The Costs

Fees for facial plastic surgery vary widely and depend on the individual surgeon, the complexity of the procedure, and where the surgery is being done. Your facial plastic surgeon and his staff will discuss costs with you before you decide to proceed.

Surgery that is done for cosmetic reasons usually is considered elective and is not covered by insurance. Full or partial coverage may be granted when there is a functional reason for the surgery. This may apply to orthognathic surgery, some types of rhinoplasty, and certain reconstructive procedures. You should consult your insurance company representative in advance to determine whether your company will consider a claim. Those expenses that are not covered by insurance can be taken as an itemized tax deduction.

Most facial plastic surgeons require payment in advance. If procedures are not covered by insurance, ask about other payment options. A growing number of surgeons, for example, accept payment by major credit card. A few have special loan plans with area banks.